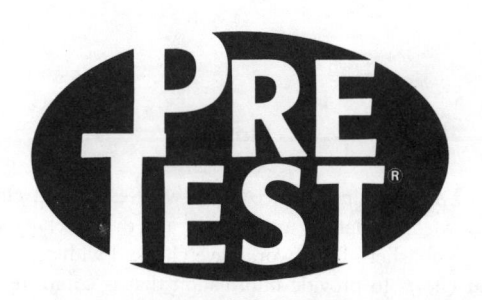

Psychiatry
PreTest® Self-Assessment and Review

Notice

Medicine is an ever-changing science. As new research and clinical experience broaden our knowledge, changes in treatment and drug therapy are required. The authors and the publisher of this work have checked with sources believed to be reliable in their efforts to provide information that is complete and generally in accord with the standards accepted at the time of publication. However, in view of the possibility of human error or changes in medical sciences, neither the authors nor the publisher nor any other party who has been involved in the preparation or publication of this work warrants that the information contained herein is in every respect accurate or complete, and they disclaim all responsibility for any errors or omissions or for the results obtained from use of the information contained in this work. Readers are encouraged to confirm the information contained herein with other sources. For example and in particular, readers are advised to check the product information sheet included in the package of each drug they plan to administer to be certain that the information contained in this work is accurate and that changes have not been made in the recommended dose or in the contraindications for administration. This recommendation is of particular importance in connection with new or infrequently used drugs.

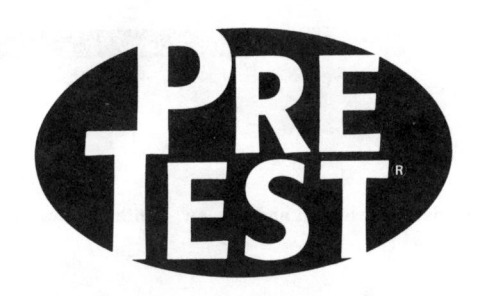

Psychiatry
PreTest® Self-Assessment and Review
Tenth Edition

Debra L. Klamen, M.D., M.H.P.E., F.A.P.A.
Associate Professor of Psychiatry
Director, Undergraduate Medical Education in Psychiatry
Assistant Dean for Preclerkship Curriculum
University of Illinois at Chicago College of Medicine
Chicago, Illinois

Philip Pan, M.D.
Clinical Assistant Professor
Department of Psychiatry
University of Illinois at Chicago College of Medicine
Chicago, Illinois

Staff Forensic Psychiatrist
Forensic Clinical Services of the Circuit Court of Cook County
Chicago, Illinois

Staff Psychiatrist
Du Page County Health Department, Crisis and Access Center
Lombard, Illinois

McGraw Hill

Boston   Burr Ridge, IL   Dubuque, IA   Madison, WI   New York
San Francisco   St. Louis   Bangkok   Bogotá   Caracas   Kuala Lumpur   Lisbon
London   Madrid   Mexico City   Milan   Montreal   New Delhi   Santiago
Seoul   Singapore   Sydney   Taipei   Toronto

Psychiatry: PreTest Self-Assessment and Review, Tenth Edition
International Edition 2004

Exclusive rights by McGraw-Hill Education (Asia), for manufacture and export. This book cannot be re-exported from the country to which it is sold by McGraw-Hill. The International Edition is not available in North America.

Copyright © 2004 by The **McGraw-Hill Companies**, Inc. All rights reserved. Except as permitted under the United States Copyright Act of 1976, no part of this publication may be reproduced or distributed in any form or by any means, or stored in a database or retrieval system, without the prior written consent of publisher, including, but not limited to, in any network or other electronic storage or transmission, or broadcast for distance learning.

Some ancillaries, including electronic and print components, may not be available to customers outside the United States.

10 09 08 07 06 05 04 03 02 01
20 09 08 07 06 05 04
FC CMO

Library of Congress Cataloging-in-Publication Data

Klamen, Debra L.
    Psychiatry : PreTest self-assessment and review.—10th ed. / Debra L. Klamen, Philip Pan ; student reviews, Alan S. Anschel, Adam Landman, Christopher T. Lang.
    p. ; cm.
    Rev. ed of: Psychiatry / Giulia Mancini-Mezzacappa. 9th ed. c2001.
    Includes bibliographical references.
    ISBN 007-138919-9
    1. Psychiatry—Examinations, questions, etc. I. Mancini-Mezzacappa, Giulia. Psychiatry. II. Pan, Philip. III. Title.
    [DNLM: 1. Mental Disorders—Examination Questions. 2. Psychotherapy—Examination Questions. WM 18.2 K63p 2003]
    RC457.M365 2003
    616.89'0076—dc21   2003044529

When ordering this title, use ISBN 007-123591-4

Printed in Singapore

Student Reviewers

Alan S. Anschel
University of Medicine and Dentistry of New Jersey
Robert Wood Johnson Medical School
Piscataway, New Jersey
Class of 2004

Adam Landman
University of Medicine and Dentistry of New Jersey
Robert Wood Johnson Medical School
Piscataway, New Jersey
Class of 2004

Christopher T. Lang
State University of New York-Buffalo
Buffalo, New York
Class of 2002

Contents

Introduction ix

Evaluation, Assessment, and Diagnosis
Questions 1
Answers, Explanations, and References 16

Human Behavior: Theories of Personality and Development
Questions 31
Answers, Explanations, and References 44

Human Behavior: Biologic and Related Sciences
Questions 59
Answers, Explanations, and References 70

Disorders of Childhood and Adolescence
Questions 79
Answers, Explanations, and References 85

Cognitive Disorders and Consultation-Liaison Psychiatry
Questions 91
Answers, Explanations, and References 109

Schizophrenia and Other Psychotic Disorders
Questions 125
Answers, Explanations, and References 138

Psychotherapies
Questions 147
Answers, Explanations, and References 161

Mood Disorders
Questions 175
Answers, Explanations, and References 185

Anxiety, Somatoform, and Dissociative Disorders
Questions 193
Answers, Explanations, and References 201

Personality Disorders, Human Sexuality, and Miscellaneous Syndromes
Questions 207
Answers, Explanations, and References 221

Substance-Related Disorders
Questions 231
Answers, Explanations, and References 241

Psychopharmacology and Other Somatic Therapies
Questions 249
Answers, Explanations, and References 269

Law and Ethics in Psychiatry
Questions 283
Answers, Explanations, and References 289

Bibliography 295
Index 297

Introduction

Psychiatry: PreTest® Self-Assessment and Review, Tenth Edition, has been designed to provide medical students, psychiatric residents, psychiatrists, mental health professionals, and international medical graduates with a comprehensive and convenient instrument for self-assessment and review. The 500 questions provided have been designed to parallel the topics, format, and degree of difficulty of the questions contained in the United States Medical Licensing Examination (USMLE) Step 1.

Each question in the book is accompanied by an answer, a paragraph explanation, and a specific page reference to a standard textbook or other major resource. These books have been carefully selected for their educational excellence and ready availability in most libraries. A bibliography that lists all the sources used in the book follows the last chapter. Diagnostic nomenclature is that of the fourth edition of *Diagnostic and Statistical Manual of Mental Disorders* (DSM-IV).

One effective way to use this book is to allow yourself one minute to answer each question in a given chapter and to mark your answer beside the question. By following this suggestion, you will be training yourself for the time limits commonly imposed by examinations.

Since there are few absolutes in clinical practice, remember to simply choose the best possible answer. There are no "trick" questions intended. Rather, each question has been designed to address a significant topic. Some important topics are deliberately duplicated in other sections of the book when this is deemed helpful. All questions apply to the treatment of adults unless otherwise indicated.

When you have finished answering the questions in a chapter, you should then spend as much time as you need to verify your answers and to absorb the explanations. Although you should pay special attention to the explanations for the questions you answered incorrectly, you should read every explanation. Each explanation is designed to reinforce and supplement the information tested by the question. When you identify a gap in your fund of knowledge, or if you simply need more information about a topic, you should consult and study the references indicated.

Evaluation, Assessment, and Diagnosis

Questions

DIRECTIONS: Each item below contains a question or incomplete statement followed by suggested responses. Select the **one best** response to each question.

1. A 42-year-old man comes to the emergency room with the chief complaint that "the men are following me." He also complains of hearing a voice telling him to hurt others. He tells the examiner that the news anchorman gives him special messages about the state of the world every night through the TV. This last belief is an example of which of the following psychiatric findings?
   a. Grandiose delusion
   b. Illusion
   c. Loose association
   d. Idea of reference
   e. Clouding of consciousness

2. A 32-year-old woman is seen in an outpatient psychiatric clinic for the chief complaint of a depressed mood for 4 months. During the interview, she gives very long, complicated explanations and many unnecessary details before finally answering the original questions. This style of train of thought is an example of which psychiatric finding?
   a. Loose association
   b. Circumstantiality
   c. Neologism
   d. Perseveration
   e. Flight of ideas

3. Which of the following is the best definition of a delusion?
   a. Fixed false belief
   b. Perceptual misrepresentation of a sensory image
   c. Perceptual representation of a sound or an image not actually present
   d. Pathological self-preoccupation
   e. Dissociative fugue

2 Psychiatry

4. A 55-year-old man is brought to the psychiatrist by his wife after she found him wandering outside of their home wearing only his underwear. On exam, the patient notes that his memory is "not as good as it used to be." Which of the following tests is most likely to be helpful in the diagnosis of this patient?
a. EEG
b. MRI
c. Serum glucose
d. Serum amylase
e. Urinary myoglobin

5. A 56-year-old man has been hospitalized for a myocardial infarction. Two days after admission, he awakens in the middle of the night and screams that there is a man standing by the window in his room. When the nurse enters the room and turns on a light, the patient is relieved to learn that the "man" was a drape by the window. This misperception of reality is best described by which psychiatric term?
a. Delusion
b. Hallucination
c. Illusion
d. Projection
e. Synesthesia

Items 6–7

6. A 1-year-old girl is brought to the physician by her mother. The child had been developing normally until about 6 to 9 months of age. At 9 months, her mother noticed that the girl's head growth had begun to decelerate, she seemed "floppy," and she had lost interest in playing. She had recently been noted to have episodes of crying, screaming, and intense hyperactivity. Which of the following diagnoses is most likely?
a. Asperger's disorder
b. Down syndrome
c. Congenital rubella
d. Rett's disorder
e. Childhood disintegrative disorder

7. According to the *DSM-IV-TR*, which category does this child's diagnosis fall under?
a. Pervasive developmental disorders
b. Mental retardation
c. Psychotic disorders
d. Learning disorders
e. Disruptive behavior disorders

8. A psychiatric resident is called to consult on a 75-year-old woman who underwent a hip replacement 2 days before. On examination, the resident notes that the patient states the date is 1956, and she thinks she is at her son's house. These impairments illustrate which aspect of the mental status examination?
a. Concentration
b. Memory
c. Thought process
d. Orientation
e. Level of consciousness

9. A 52-year-old man is sent to see a psychiatrist after he is disciplined at his job because he consistently turns in his assignments late. He states he is not about to turn in anything until it is "perfect, unlike all of my colleagues." He has few friends, because he annoys them with his demands for "precise timeliness" and because of his lack of emotional warmth. This has been a lifelong pattern of behavior for the patient, though he refuses to believe the problems have anything to do with his personal behavior. Which of the following is this patient's most likely diagnosis?
a. Obsessive-compulsive disorder
b. Obsessive-compulsive personality disorder
c. Borderline personality disorder
d. Bipolar disorder, mixed state
e. Anxiety disorder not otherwise specified

10. A 23-year-old woman works in a supervised workshop. She can schedule her own daily activities and tell time. She cannot cook her own meals without supervision, nor can she make change for a dollar. Which of the following levels of mentation does this patient fall into?

a. Normal IQ
b. Mild mental retardation
c. Moderate mental retardation
d. Severe mental retardation
e. Profound mental retardation

11. A 22-year-old man comes to the emergency room with the chief complaint that "people are all against me." During the interview, he is hypervigilant about his surroundings and suspicious of the examiner. Suddenly, in the middle of the interview, the patient clenches his jaw and both his fists, then stands up. Which of the following is the best action for the interviewer to take next?

a. Tell the patient to sit down immediately
b. Continue to sit calmly until the patient sits too
c. Reassure the patient by touching him on the shoulder
d. Stand up slowly and inform the patient that no one will hurt him
e. Put the patient in leather restraints and give him haloperidol

Items 12–13

12. A 23-year-old woman comes to the emergency room with the chief complaint of hearing voices for 7 months. Besides the hallucinations, she has the idea that the radio is giving her special messages. When asked the meaning of the proverb "People in glass houses should not throw stones," the patient replies, "Because the windows would break." Which mental status finding does this patient display?

a. Poverty of content
b. Concrete thinking
c. Flight of ideas
d. Loose associations
e. Autistic thinking

13. Which of the following diagnoses is most likely?
a. Dysthymic disorder
b. Schizophreniform disorder
c. Schizoid personality disorder
d. Communication disorder
e. Schizophrenia

14. A 69-year-old man is brought to see his physician by his wife. She notes that over the past year he has had a slow stepwise decline in his cognitive functioning. One year ago she felt his thinking was "as good as it always was," but now he gets lost around the house and can't remember simple directions. The patient states he feels fine, though he is depressed about his loss of memory. He is eating and sleeping well. Which of the following diagnoses is most likely?
a. Multi-infarct dementia
b. Mood disorder secondary to a general medical condition
c. Schizoaffective disorder
d. Delirium
e. Major depression

15. A 50-year-old woman becomes depressed after her son dies in a car crash. She and her husband are devastated by the loss. Although the patient has been in otherwise good health, she has lost 10 lb in the last 2 months. She tells the physician that she would be better off dead. Which of the following statements with regard to the assessment of suicide risk in this patient is true?
a. The patient's gender puts her at higher risk for a completed suicide than if she were male
b. The patient is unlikely to commit suicide because she was able to talk about it
c. The patient's age puts her at higher risk than a younger (<40 years old) patient
d. The patient's good health puts her at higher risk for a successful attempt at suicide
e. The patient's marital status puts her at higher risk of suicide than if she were single

6   Psychiatry

16. A 45-year-old man is in chronic liver failure and is being evaluated for his suitability to be put on the transplant list. The psychiatrist doing the evaluation would like to administer a psychological test to screen for serious psychopathology and to ascertain the patient's likely response to medical intervention. Which of the following tests is most likely to be helpful in this instance?

a. Minnesota Multiphasic Personality Inventory (MMPI)
b. Symptom Checklist-90-Revised (SCL-90-R)
c. Wisconsin card sorting test
d. Strong Vocational Interest Bank (SVIB)
e. Structured Clinical Interview for Diagnosis Revised (SCIDR)

17. During a psychoeducational evaluation, a school psychologist shows a 10-year-old girl a series of cards with ambiguous pictures on them and asks her to make up her own stories about what is happening in each one. Which of the following tests is described above?

a. Trail-making test
b. California verbal learning test
c. Thematic apperception test (TAT)
d. Vineland Adaptive Behavior Scales
e. Wechsler Intelligence Scale for Children III (WISC-III)

Items 18–19

18. A 24-year-old man is admitted to the inpatient psychiatry unit after his mother noted he was standing in place for hours at a time in abnormal postures. On exam, the patient is standing in the examining room with one arm raised directly above his head and the other straight out in front of him. He is mute, does not appear aware of his surroundings, and actively resists any attempts to change his position. Which of the following best describes the patient's behavior?

a. Apraxia
b. Dystonia
c. Synesthesia
d. Catatonia
e. Trance state

19. This symptom can be seen in which of the following diagnoses?
a. Schizophrenia
b. Delirium
c. Parkinson's disease
d. Neuroleptic malignant syndrome
e. Huntington's disease

20. A psychiatrist is seeing a patient in his outpatient practice. The patient treats the psychiatrist as if he were unreliable and punitive, though he had not been either. The patient's father was an alcoholic who often did not show up to pick her up from school and frequently hit her. The psychiatrist begins to feel as if he must over-protect the patient and treat her gingerly, much like he treated his younger sister when she was small. The psychiatrist's behavior is an example of which psychological mechanism?
a. Reaction formation
b. Projection
c. Countertransference
d. Identification with the aggressor
e. Illusion

21. A 36-year-old woman with schizophrenia comes to the emergency room with the chief complaint that "they are trying to kill me." In the examining room, she is hypervigilant and insists on sitting in the corner with her back to the wall. Suddenly she begins to stare intently into the corner and say, "No, you can't make me do that!" Which of the following symptoms is this patient most likely experiencing?
a. Concrete thinking
b. Depersonalization
c. Flight of ideas
d. Hallucination
e. Idea of reference

8　Psychiatry

22. A patient is able to appreciate subtle nuances in thinking and can use metaphors and understand them. This patient's thinking can be best defined by which of the following terms?
a. Intellectualization
b. Abstract
c. Rationalization
d. Concrete
e. Isolation of affect

23. A 65-year-old man, who was hospitalized for an acute pneumonia 3 days previously, begins screaming for his nurse, stating that "there are people in the room out to get me." He then gets out of bed and begins pulling out his intravenous line. On exam, he alternates between agitation and somnolence. He is not oriented to time or place. His vital signs are: pulse, 126/min; respiration, 32/min; blood pressure, 80/58; temperature, 102.5°F. Which of the following diagnoses best fits this patient's clinical picture?
a. Dementia
b. Schizophreniform disorder
c. Fugue state
d. Delirium
e. Brief psychotic episode

24. A 35-year-old man is brought to see a psychiatrist by his wife, who states her husband keeps getting lost, even in places he has been familiar with for years. The patient's father was institutionalized and died at age 37. On exam, the patient is oriented to person only. He cannot accurately make change for a dollar, though he used to work as a banker. Which of the following diagnostic tests would be most useful for this patient?
a. EEG
b. Liver function tests
c. Serum amylase
d. Blood toxicology screen
e. MRI

25. A 34-year-old woman comes to her physician with the chief complaint of a depressed mood. She also notes trouble concentrating, hypersomnia, a 20-lb weight gain, and slowed mentation. Which of the following diagnostic tests will be most helpful in diagnosing this patient?

a. Thyroid function tests
b. Liver function tests
c. Serum ceruloplasmin
d. EEG
e. Urine amino acids

26. A 23-year-old man presents to the emergency room with the history of a fever up to 100.5°F intermittently over the past 2 weeks, a persistent cough, and a 10-lb weight loss in the past month. He notes that he has also been becoming increasingly forgetful for the past month, and that his thinking is "not always clear." He has gotten lost twice recently while driving. Which of the following diagnostic tests will be most helpful with this patient?

a. EEG
b. Liver function tests
c. Thyroid function tests
d. HIV antibody test
e. Skull x-ray

27. A 27-year-old woman comes to her physician with the chief complaint of passing out several times in the past 3 weeks. The patient states that she does not remember what happens, but suddenly she "wakes up on the floor." Her husband states that each of these episodes has occurred in the middle of a fight between the two. He notes that his wife will suddenly crumple to the floor, "jerk all over," and remain that way for approximately 5 min. When she wakes up, he states she is fully alert and oriented. Which of the following diagnostic tests will be most helpful with this patient?

a. EEG
b. ECG
c. MRI
d. Dexamethasone suppression test
e. Serum amylase

Psychiatry

28. A 19-year-old woman presents to the emergency room with the chief complaint of a depressed mood for 2 weeks. She states that since her therapist went on vacation she has noted suicidal ideation, crying spells, and an increased appetite. She states that she has left 40 messages on the therapist's answering machine, telling him she is going to kill herself, and that it would serve him right for leaving her. On physical exam, multiple well-healed scars and cigarette burns are noted on the anterior aspect of both forearms. Which of the following diagnoses best fits this patient's clinical presentation?

a. Dysthymic disorder
b. Bipolar disorder
c. Panic disorder
d. Borderline personality disorder
e. Schizoaffective disorder

29. A 28-year-old man comes to the physician with the chief complaint of having been depressed for years. He notes that his mood is never good, though he has never seriously considered suicide. He often feels hopeless and has problems concentrating. His sleep and appetite have not changed. He denies hallucinations of any kind. Which of the following diagnoses best fit this patient's clinical picture?

a. Conversion disorder
b. Avoidant personality disorder
c. Dysthymic disorder
d. Major depression
e. Adjustment disorder

30. A 29-year-old man is brought to the emergency room by his wife after he woke up with paralysis of his right arm. The patient states that the day before, he had gotten into a verbal altercation with his mother over her intrusiveness into his life. The patient notes he has always had mixed feelings about his mother, but that people should always respect their mothers above all else. Which of the following diagnoses best fits this patient's clinical picture?

a. Major depression
b. Conversion disorder
c. Histrionic personality disorder
d. Fugue state
e. Adjustment disorder

31. A 28-year-old business executive comes to see her physician because she is having difficulty in her new position, as it requires her to do frequent public speaking. She states she is terrified that she will do or say something that will cause her extreme embarrassment. The patient says that when she must speak in public, she becomes extremely anxious and her heart beats uncontrollably. Which of the following diagnoses best fits this patient's clinical picture?

a. Panic disorder
b. Avoidant personality disorder
c. Specific phobia
d. Agoraphobia
e. Social phobia

32. A 24-year-old male comes to the physician with the chief complaint that his nose is too big to the point of being hideous. The patient states his nose is a constant embarrassment to him and he would like it surgically reduced. He tells the physician that three previous surgeons had all refused to operate on him because they said his nose was fine, but the patient states that "they just didn't want such a difficult case." The physician observes that the patient's nose is of normal size and shape. Which of the following diagnoses best fits this patient's clinical picture?

a. Schizophrenia
b. Narcissistic personality disorder
c. Body dysmorphic disorder
d. Anxiety disorder not otherwise specified
e. Schizoaffective disorder

Items 33–34

33. Prenatal care, stress reduction seminars, and lead elimination laws are all examples of which kind of program?

a. Primary prevention
b. Secondary prevention
c. Tertiary prevention
d. Case management
e. Outpatient commitment

34. A medical student chooses psychiatry as a career because he wants to devote his career to the treatment of mental illness before it causes permanent disability. This type of work is best defined by which term?
a. Case management
b. Long-term care
c. Primary prevention
d. Secondary prevention
e. Tertiary prevention

35. Which of the following terms best fits the definition, "The proportion of a population affected by a disorder at a given time"?
a. Prevalence
b. Incidence
c. Validity
d. Reliability
e. Relative risk

36. A diagnostic test has a sensitivity of 64% and a specificity of 99%. Such a test would carry the risk of which kind of problem?
a. High relative risk
b. Low likelihood ratio
c. False negatives
d. False positives
e. Low power

37. A 29-year-old woman comes to the emergency room with the chief complaint of a depressed mood for 3 weeks. As she is telling the physician about this, she smiles broadly. Which of the following best describes this behavior?
a. Incongruent affect
b. Perseveration
c. Disorientation
d. Flight of ideas
e. Word salad

38. A 56-year-old man is brought to the physician's office by his wife because she has noted a personality change in the past 3 months. While the patient is being interviewed, he answers every question with the same three words. Which of the following symptoms best fits this patient's behavior?

a. Negative symptoms
b. Disorientation
c. Concrete thinking
d. Perseveration
e. Circumstantiality

39. A 32-year-old patient is being interviewed in his physician's office. He responds to each question, but he gives long answers with a great deal of tedious and unnecessary detail. Which of the following symptoms best describes this patient's presentation?

a. Blocking
b. Tangentiality
c. Circumstantiality
d. Looseness of associations
e. Flight of ideas

40. An 18-year-old man is brought to the emergency room by the police after he is found walking along the edge of a high building. In the emergency room, he is noted to mumble to himself and appears to be responding to internal stimuli. When asked open-ended questions, he suddenly stops his answer in the middle of a sentence, as if he has forgotten what to say. Which of the following symptoms best describes this last behavior?

a. Incongruent affect
b. Blocking
c. Perseveration
d. Tangentiality
e. Thought insertion

41. A 26-year-old woman with panic disorder notes that during the middle of one of her attacks she feels as if she is disconnected from the world, as if it is unreal or distant. Which of the following terms best describes this symptom?

a. Dulled perception
b. Illusion
c. Retardation of thought
d. Depersonalization
e. Derealization

42. A patient with a chronic psychotic disorder is convinced that she has caused a recent earthquake because she was bored and wishing for something exciting to occur. Which of the following symptoms most closely describes this patient's thoughts?

a. Thought broadcasting
b. Magical thinking
c. Echolalia
d. Nihilism
e. Obsession

43. A 43-year-old man tells his psychiatrist that he is spending several hours in the morning checking all the light switches to make sure they are off. He states that if he does not do this he is overcome with anxiety. This is an example of which of the following symptoms?

a. Catalepsy
b. Compulsions
c. Magical thinking
d. Anhedonia
e. Folie à deux

44. A 45-year-old man with a chronic psychotic disorder is interviewed after his admission to a psychiatric unit. He mimics the examiner's body posture and movements during the interview. Which of the following terms best characterizes this patient's symptom?

a. Folie à deux
b. Dereistic thinking
c. Echolalia
d. Echopraxia
e. Fugue

DIRECTIONS: Each group of questions below consists of lettered options followed by a set of numbered items. For each numbered item, select the **one** lettered option with which it is **most** closely associated. Each lettered option may be used once, more than once, or not at all.

Items 45–47

Match the patient's symptoms with the appropriate diagnostic axis.
a. Axis I
b. Axis II
c. Axis III
d. Axis IV
e. Axis V

45. A 32-year-old man complains of depressed mood, poor concentration, a 25-lb weight gain, and hypersomnia. He is subsequently diagnosed with hypothyroidism. **(CHOOSE 1 AXIS)**

46. A 46-year-old college professor has not been able to go to work for the past 6 weeks because of severe depression and suicidal ideation. **(CHOOSE 1 AXIS)**

47. A 23-year-old woman works in a sheltered workshop. She is unable to make change for a dollar or read beyond a second-grade level. She has a genetic makeup of 47 chromosomes with three copies of chromosome 21. **(CHOOSE 1 AXIS)**

Evaluation, Assessment, and Diagnosis

Answers

1. The answer is d. *(Kaplan, 8/e, pp 252, 285.)* An idea of reference is the belief that an object, event, or person in one's environment (commonly the television or radio) has particular personal significance. A delusion is a fixed, false belief, and a grandiose delusion has a theme that attributes special powers or talents to the delusional person. An illusion is the misperception or misinterpretation of real external sensory stimuli. A loose association describes a disturbance in the continuity of thought in which ideas expressed do not seem to be logically related. Clouding of consciousness refers to an overall reduced awareness of the surrounding environment.

2. The answer is b. *(Kaplan, 8/e, pp 252, 282.)* Circumstantiality indicates the loss of a goal-directed thought process: the patient brings in many irrelevant details and comments, but eventually will get back to the point. A neologism is a fabricated word made up by the patient, usually a combination of other existing words. Perseveration, often associated with cognitive disorders, refers to a response that persists even after a new stimulus has been introduced—for example, a patient asked to repeat the phrase "no ifs, ands, or buts" responds by saying, "no ifs, ifs, ifs, ifs." Flight of ideas is a disorder of thinking in which the patient expresses thoughts very rapidly, with constant shifting from one idea to another, though the ideas are often connected.

3. The answer is a. *(Kaplan, 8/e, pp 252, 283, 665.)* A delusion is a fixed, false belief that is not in keeping with a patient's cultural background. The perceptual misrepresentation of a real sensory image is an illusion. The perceptual representation of a sound or an image that is not actually present is a hallucination. A pathological self-preoccupation is the definition of egomania. A dissociative fugue is a state in which patients travel away from their homes or work and assume new identities or occupations while forgetting important aspects and details of their former lives.

4. The answer is b. (*Kaplan, 8/e, pp 264–266. Stoudemire, 3/e, pp 137–138.*) An MRI may be helpful in ruling out organic causes of an apparent dementia, especially tumors or subcortical arteriosclerotic encephalopathy. An EEG is not sensitive for detecting dementia—it is often normal in the early and middle stages. (It is, however, quite sensitive for detecting delirium.) Very low or high serum glucose levels can be associated with delirium, and hypoglycemia is also associated with panic attacks, anxiety, or depression, but not dementia. Serum amylase may be increased in bulimia nervosa. Increased urine myoglobin is seen in neuroleptic malignant syndrome, in a variety of drug intoxications, and in patients in restraints.

5. The answer is c. (*Kaplan, 8/e, pp 220, 282–284.*) An illusion is the misperception or misinterpretation of a real sensory stimulus, as opposed to a hallucination, which is a false sensory perception unrelated to any real sensory stimulus. A delusion is a fixed, false belief that is unrelated to a patient's intelligence or cultural background. By definition, a delusion cannot be corrected with the use of logic or reasoning. Projection is a defense mechanism in which the patient reacts to an inner unacceptable impulse as if it were outside the self. For example, a paranoid patient reacts to others as if they are going to hurt him. This is because the patient's unacceptable hostile impulses are projected onto others and the patient reacts as if the others have hostile impulses of their own toward the patient. Synesthesia is a sensation or hallucination caused by another sensation (for example, a visual sensation triggers the hallucination of an auditory sensation).

6. The answer is d. (*Ebert, pp 546–556.*) Patients diagnosed with Rett's disorder have normal prenatal and postnatal development but, between ages 5 to 30 months, they begin to lose previously acquired purposeful hand skills and develop stereotyped hand movements (hand wringing or hand washing) and poorly coordinated gait or trunk movements. These patients have severe to profound mental retardation and severe receptive and expressive language deficits. They also lose all interest in social interaction. Characteristically, head circumference is normal at birth, but between 5 months and 4 years of age the rate of the head growth decelerates rapidly. Rett's disorder has been described only in females and is very rare.

7. The answer is a. (*Ebert, pp 546–556, 565.*) Rett's disorder is one of the pervasive developmental disorders, along with autistic disorder, Asperger's disorder, and childhood disintegrative disorder (a catastrophic deterioration of cognitive functions, social awareness, and adaptive behavior that starts after 2 years of normal development).

8. The answer is d. *(Kaplan, 8/e, pp 250–254.)* Orientation refers to the state of awareness of the individual as to time and place, and to the awareness of the identity of oneself and others in the environment. This is the reason patients' cognitive states are often referred to as "oriented × 3," meaning oriented to person, place, and time.

9. The answer is b. *(Kaplan, 8/e, p 775.)* The essential feature of obsessive-compulsive personality disorder is a preoccupation with perfection, orderliness, and control. Individuals with this disorder lose the main point of an activity and miss deadlines because they pay too much attention to rules and details and are not satisfied with anything less than "perfection." As in other personality disorders, symptoms are ego-syntonic and create interpersonal, social, and occupational difficulties. Obsessive-compulsive disorder is differentiated from obsessive-compulsive personality disorder by the presence of obsessions and compulsions. Patients with borderline personality disorder present with a history of pervasive instability of mood, relationships, and self-image beginning by early adulthood. Their behavior is often impulsive and self-damaging. Patients with bipolar disorder present with problems with mood stability; mood may be depressed for several weeks at a time, then euphoric. Patients with an anxiety disorder not otherwise specified present with anxiety as a main symptom, though they do not specifically fit any other more specific anxiety disorder as per *DSM-IV-TR*.

10. The answer is c. *(Ebert, p 546.)* Patients with moderate mental retardation (MR) are generally able to work in structured competitive or sheltered workshop settings. While they can perform basic activities of daily living (getting dressed, eating with utensils, telling time, and making schedules for themselves), they are unable to make change for a dollar, use public transportation, or cook meals unsupervised. They usually require custodial supervision.

11. The answer is d. *(Stoudemire, 3/e, pp 697–699.)* A patient seen in an emergency room setting with prominent symptoms of paranoia ("people are all against me," hypervigilence, suspiciousness) should be watched closely, since the paranoia often extends to the environment in which the patient finds him- or herself. Signs of impending violence include the clenching of jaw or fists and increasing agitation (standing up, increased pacing, raised voice). The physician should not take a demanding tone with this kind of patient nor touch him or her. Standing as the patient stands ensures that the examiner is not at a physical disadvantage or vulnerable position as the patient stands. Reassuring the patient directly in a slow, even tone of voice that no one will hurt him or her may often allow the patient to relax somewhat, avoiding the need for full leather restraints or haloperidol.

12. The answer is b. *(Kaplan, 8/e, pp 251–252.)* Patients who present with concrete thinking have lost the ability to form abstract concepts, such as metaphors, and focus instead on actual things and facts. Concrete thinking is the norm in children and is seen in cognitive disorders (mental retardation, dementia) and schizophrenia.

13. The answer is e. *(Kaplan, 8/e, p 481.)* Hearing voices for 7 months, having ideas of reference, and displaying concrete abstract interpretation on exam all point to a likely diagnosis of schizophrenia. Key features of schizophrenia include at least two psychotic symptoms (hallucinations, delusions, evidence of a thought disorder, disorganized or catatonic behavior, or negative symptoms) present for at least 1 month; impairment in social or occupational functioning; duration of at least 6 months; symptoms not due to either a mood disorder or a medical or substance-induced disorder. Schizophreniform patients must fulfill all the same criteria except that the duration of illness is less than 6 months.

14. The answer is a. *(Ebert, p 216.)* Multiple cerebral infarcts cause a progressive dementia (usually described as stepwise), focal neurological signs, and often neuropsychiatric symptoms such as depression, mood lability (but usually not elated mood), and delusions. Loose associations, catatonic posturing, and bizarre proverb interpretations occurring with affective symptoms are typical of schizoaffective disorder. In delirium, one would expect to see the waxing and waning of consciousness over time, including problems with orientation to person, place, and time.

15. The answer is c. (*Stoudemire, 3/e, p 707.*) Males have a higher risk of completed suicide than do females (though females attempt suicide more frequently). People who commit suicide usually talk about their intent with others before going ahead with their plans. People over 45 are at higher risk than younger people. Good health lowers the risk for suicide, and poor health increases it. People who live with others or are married are less at risk of committing suicide than people who live alone.

16. The answer is a. (*Stoudemire, 3/e, pp 96–109.*) Three instruments are used to assess patients' functioning: psychological tests, rating scales, and structured interviews. Psychological tests use questions or statements patients have to agree or disagree with, or similar sampling methods, to obtain more information about individuals' cognitive functions, emotional status, expectations, beliefs, and many other areas that are significant in psychiatry. Answers are standardized to ensure reliability. Psychological tests are helpful tools because they can provide understanding of personality traits, symptoms, and cognitive deficits not readily accessible during an unstructured evaluation. A diagnosis should not be made only on the basis of test results. Commonly used psychological tests are the Wechsler Adult Intelligence Scale (WAIS), the MMPI, and projective tests such as the Rorschach inkblot test. Rating scales are standardized devices that allow an observer to rate the patient's behavior in specific areas. An example is the SCL-90-R, used to ascertain which symptoms might be occurring in a given patient. In semistructured interviews, questions are predetermined and responses are formulated in a way that permits standardization (yes/no, not at all/sometimes/always, and so on). The SCIDR is an example of this kind of test. It is used to determine the *DSM-IV* diagnosis in the patient being examined. The Wisconsin card sorting test assesses abstract reasoning and flexibility in problem solving. The SVIB is a test administered to help determine the possible vocational interests of the subject. It is sometimes given to students in high schools.

The MMPI and MMPI-2 (a revised version) are among the most used psychological tests. They are called personality tests because they provide information about the patient's characterological traits in addition to information concerning the patient's symptoms. The MMPI consists of a 566-item checklist in a true/false format, to be completed by the patient in one to two hours. The questions are worded so that a person with an elementary education would not have difficulty understanding them and are constructed to explore the presence or absence of emotions, experiences, and thoughts. The items are divided into groups, each intended to provide information in one of nine clinical scales: hypochondriasis, depression, hysteria, psychopathic deviance, masculinity-femininity, paranoia, psychoasthenia, schizophrenia, and mania. The patient's responses are computer scored, and the patient's profile (personality) depends on the score in each scale. For example, a patient with a high score in the schizophrenia scale will typically emerge as distrustful, keeping people at a distance, using projection as a main defense, and so on.

17. The answer is c. *(Stoudemire, 3/e, p 101.)* The TAT, a projective test, consists of 30 pictures representing a particular scene or interpersonal situation and one blank card. In response to each card, the patient is asked to make up a story about what is being depicted in the card, and the examiner records these responses verbatim. The TAT is used to investigate the psychodynamics of the patient with regard to interpersonal relationships via the manner in which the patient interprets the various environments depicted in the cards. The Trail-making test assesses motor speed, visuomotor tracking, and attention. Part A asks the patient to draw lines to connect consecutively numbered circles on a worksheet, and part B asks the patient to connect consecutively numbered and lettered circles by alternating between the two sequences. The California verbal learning test assesses retention, recognition, and recall in the verbal memory system by asking subjects to learn new orally presented material, retain this information in short- and long-term memory, and recall the information in the context of semantic cues. The Weschler Intelligence Scale for Children is an instrument used to measure intelligence, and the Vineland Adaptive Behavior Scales measure the developmental level of adaptive functioning.

18. The answer is d. *(Ebert, p 262.)* The voluntary assumption of an inappropriate or bizarre posture for long periods of time is called catatonic posturing and is usually seen in schizophrenia, especially of the catatonic type. In catatonic posturing, patients resist attempts to make them change position (this is also called negativism). A similar symptom, waxy flexibility, refers to patients that maintain the body position into which they are placed. Apraxia refers to the inability to perform voluntary motor activity in the absence of motor or sensory deficits. Dystonia refers to the protracted contraction of a group of muscles. In synesthesia, the stimulation of one sensory modality produces a sensation belonging to another sensory modality (e.g., a color is perceived as a smell). Trance is a sleeplike condition characterized by a reduced state of consciousness.

19. The answer is a. *(Ebert, p 262.)* Although Parkinson's disease, Neuroleptic malignant syndrome, and Huntington's disease can all present with motor abnormalities, schizophrenia is the only choice in the question that may present with catatonia.

20. The answer is c. *(Ebert, p 113.)* Countertransference is the name given to the analyst's or psychotherapist's transference response to the patient. As with patients' transference, the particular form the countertransference takes depends on the therapist's past experiences, relationships, and unresolved conflicts. As with transference, countertransference is not limited to the patient-therapist relationship, but may be present in any relationship. By analyzing his countertransference toward the patient, the therapist may acquire useful insight into the patient's dynamics and his own. Consequently, even negative countertransference feelings can be helpful tools in the psychotherapy process. Reaction formation, projection, and identification with the aggressor are unconscious defense mechanisms. An illusion is a perceptual misinterpretation of a real stimulus.

21. The answer is d. *(Ebert, p 261.)* A hallucination is the perception of a stimulus when no sensory stimulus is in fact present. Hallucinations can be auditory, visual, tactile, gustatory, olfactory, or kinesthetic (body movements). Auditory hallucinations are most commonly associated with psychotic illness, whereas visual, tactile, gustatory, and olfactory hallucinations often are associated with neurologic disorders. Concrete thinking is the inability to form abstract concepts, such as metaphors, and to focus instead on actual things and facts. Depersonalization is the subjective sensation of the self being disconnected from the world, unreal, or distant. Flight of ideas is a thought process in which consecutive thoughts, while related to some degree, are sequentially tangential. An idea of reference is the belief that something in the environment (commonly the TV or radio) is giving the person special messages meant only for him or her.

22. The answer is b. *(Kaplan, 8/e, p 286.)* The capacity to generalize and to formulate concepts is called abstract thinking. The inability to abstract is called concreteness and is seen in organic disorders and sometimes in schizophrenia. Abstract thinking is commonly assessed by testing similarities, differences, and the meaning of proverbs. Intellectualization, rationalization, and isolation of affect are all unconscious defenses.

23. The answer is d. *(Kaplan, 8/e, p 323.)* The patient's persecutory delusions and disorganized thinking could suggest a psychotic disorder such as schizophrenia or brief reactive psychosis, but fluctuations in consciousness and disorientation are typically found in delirium. Memory, language, and sleep-wake cycle disturbances are also typical of delirium. Delusions, hallucinations, illusions, and misperceptions are also common. The causes of delirium are many and include metabolic encephalopathies (including fever and hypoxia, as in the patient in the question), intoxications with drugs and poisons; withdrawal syndromes; head trauma; epilepsy; neoplasms; vascular disorders; allergic reactions; and injuries caused by physical agents (heat, cold, radiation).

24. The answer is e. *(Ebert, p 514.)* Huntington's disease is a progressive neurodegenerative disorder, inherited as an autosomal dominant trait, that usually manifests between 35 and 40 years of age. Affected individuals present with a progressive dementia, choreoathetoid movements, and, often, psychiatric symptoms. Computed tomography (CT) scan and nuclear magnetic resonance imaging (MRI) demonstrate gross atrophy of the putamen and the caudate.

25. The answer is a. *(Ebert, p 514.)* The woman is suffering from hypothyroidism, which frequently presents with mood symptomatology (often depression). The psychiatric picture of hypothyroidism is characterized by lethargy, mental sluggishness, and cognitive slowing. Typical physical signs and symptoms of the illness include dry skin, slow reflexes, bradycardia, nonpitting edema over the face and limbs, hair loss, and menstrual changes. Gross psychosis (myxedema madness) may also rarely be seen, in addition to the cognitive and depressive features of the disease. It is therefore essential to test the thyroid function of patients presenting with a depressed mood.

26. The answer is d. *(Stoudemire, 3/e, p 137.)* The patient has HIV-associated dementia, a disorder caused by the direct toxic effect of the HIV virus on the brain. A CD4 count below 200 is usually associated with HIV dementia, since this disorder occurs usually in the more advanced stages of AIDS. More rarely, cognitive impairments may be the first manifestation of HIV infection.

27. The answer is a. (*Stoudemire, 3/e, p 27.*) The woman has nonepileptic seizures, a form of conversion disorder. Nonepileptic seizures can often be differentiated from epileptic episodes by the presence of unusual and wild movements and vocalizations, a lack of postictal confusion, and an association with a psychosocial stressor. Sometimes the diagnosis can be made only by documenting that the behavioral manifestations of the seizure are not accompanied by epileptic activity on the EEG.

28. The answer is d. (*Ebert, p 475.*) Individuals with borderline personality disorder characteristically form intense but very unstable relationships. Since they tend to perceive themselves and others as either totally bad or perfectly good, borderline individuals either idealize or devalue any person who occupies a significant place in their lives. Usually these perceptions do not last, and the person idealized one day can be seen as completely negative the next day.

29. The answer is c. (*Ebert, p 307.*) Dysthymic disorder is characterized by a depressed mood for most of the day, for more days than not, for at least 2 years. While this mood disorder can be severe, with poor appetite, insomnia, low energy, fatigue, poor concentration, and hopelessness, the symptoms are not severe enough to meet the criteria for a major depression.

30. The answer is b. (*Ebert, p 161.*)
Conversion disorder is characterized by the sudden appearance of often dramatic neurological symptoms that are not associated with the usual diagnostic signs and test results expected for the symptoms being presented. Conversion disorder occurs in the context of a psychosocial stressor or an insoluble interpersonal or intrapsychic conflict. The psychological distress is not consciously acknowledged, but it is expressed through a metaphorical body dysfunction. In this example, the man who is torn between his duty to his mother and his intense anger at her resolved his impulse to hit her by developing a physical paralysis of his right arm.

31. The answer is e. *(Ebert, p 334.)* A social phobia is a persistent and overwhelming fear of humiliation or embarrassment in social or performance situations. This leads to high levels of distress and avoidance of those situations. Often physical symptoms of anxiety such as blushing, trembling, sweating, or tachycardia are triggered when the patient feels under evaluation or scrutiny.

32. The answer is c. *(Ebert, p 373.)* An extreme feeling of dislike for a part of the body in spite of a normal or nearly normal appearance is the main characteristic of body dysmorphic disorder. The fear of being ugly or repulsive is not decreased by reassurance and compliments and has almost a delusional quality. The social, academic, and occupational lives of individuals with this disorder are greatly affected, due to avoidance of social interactions for fear of embarrassment, the time spent in checking mirrors and seeking surgical treatment or cosmetic remedies, and the chronic emotional distress that accompanies the disorder.

33–34. The answers are 33-a, 34-d. *(Kaplan, 8/e, p 177.)* Primary prevention focuses on preventing a disorder from happening in the future and targets normal individuals at risk. The goal of secondary prevention is to address problems at an early stage to avoid future more severe problems. Tertiary prevention defines those interventions aimed at reducing the disability or the duration of a disorder in patients who are already afflicted. Case management refers to the process by which one person coordinates the efforts of the treatment team (often psychiatrists, social workers, and occupation therapists, among others) and ensures that the patient keeps appointments and complies with treatment plans. Many states have provisions for legally requiring a patient to comply with treatment outside of the hospital: this is called outpatient commitment. It is usually imposed on those patients who have a history of repeated failure to take their medication(s) as outpatients. Long-term care refers to the ability of a physician to follow a patient through all treatment modalities—emergency room, hospitalization, partial hospitalization, and outpatient treatment.

35. The answer is a. *(Kaplan, 8/e, p 174.)* Prevalence refers to the portion of the population that has a specific disorder at a specific point in time, regardless of when the disorder started. The point in time may be a date (point prevalence), a given time span (e.g., six months), or the entire life of an individual (life prevalence). The incidence of a disease refers to a rate that includes only those people who develop the disease during a specific period of time (usually 1 year). Validity refers to the accuracy and verifiability of a study. It is usually demonstrated by agreement between two attempts to measure the same issue by different methods. Reliability refers to the chance that the same experiment, done again, would have the same result: thus, the higher reliability reported, the better. Relative risk is the ratio of the incidence of a disease among people exposed to the risk factor to the incidence among those not exposed. For example, the relative risk of lung cancer is much greater for heavy smokers than for nonsmokers.

36. The answer is c. *(Kaplan, 8/e, p 175.)* Sensitivity is defined as the number of true positives divided by the sum of the number of true positives and false negatives. It is the proportion of patients with the condition in question that the test can detect. Thus, if the sensitivity is only 64%, the number of false negatives will most likely be unacceptably high.

37. The answer is a. *(Ebert, p 100.)* All the choices are elements of the mental status examination, an essential part of the psychiatric evaluation. Affect is the feeling tone that accompanies the patient's verbalizations or immediate behaviors. The interviewer's observations of the patient's affect during the whole evaluation represent an important part of the mental status evaluation. In schizophrenia, affect is often inappropriate, incongruent with the mood, or flat. Blunting of affect is also common in brain disorders. Tangentiality, circumstantiality, flight of ideas, word salad, and perseveration are forms of thought disorder. Tangentiality is present when the patient wanders and digresses to unnecessary details and the substance of the idea is not communicated. Circumstantiality is a disturbance in which the patient digresses into unnecessary details before communicating the central idea. In perseveration, the patient displays an inability to change the topic or gives the same response to different questions. In flight of ideas there are rapid, continuous verbalizations or plays on words that produce constant shifting from one idea to another. Ideas tend to be connected. In word salad, there is an incoherent mixture of words and phrases. Disorientation is an impairment of awareness of time, place, or person. A disoriented patient usually does not know the date or where he or she is. Very rarely, a person is disoriented about his or her own identity; when this symptom is present, malingering may be suspected. Disorientation is a typical finding in cognitive disorders such as delirium and dementia, but it is not usually found in primary psychotic disorders such as schizophrenia.

38. The answer is d. *(Ebert, p 106.)* Perseveration and circumstantiality are forms of thought disorder. In perseveration, the patient displays an inability to change the topic or gives the same response to different questions. Circumstantiality is a disturbance in which the patient digresses into unnecessary details before communicating the central idea. The capacity to generalize and to formulate concepts is called abstract thinking. The inability to abstract is called concreteness and is seen in organic disorders and sometimes in schizophrenia. Abstract thinking is commonly assessed by testing similarities, differences, and the meaning of proverbs. Negative symptoms include amotivation, apathy, and social withdrawal. These symptoms are often seen in schizophrenia.

39. The answer is c. *(Ebert, p 106.)* Tangentiality, circumstantiality, flight of ideas, and looseness of associations are forms of thought disorder. Tangentiality is present when the patient wanders and digresses to unnecessary details and the substance of the idea is not communicated. Circumstantiality is a disturbance in which the patient digresses into unnecessary details before communicating the central idea. In flight of ideas there are rapid, continuous verbalizations or plays on words that produce constant shifting from one idea to another. Ideas tend to be connected. In looseness of associations, the flow of thought is disconnected—ideas shift from one subject to another in a completely unrelated way.

40. The answer is b. *(Ebert, p 106.)* In blocking, the patient suddenly stops talking, usually in the middle of a sentence, and cannot complete his or her thoughts. Affect is said to be incongruent when what is observed by the examiner (affect) does not match the subjective statement of how the patient feels (mood). Perseveration is a form of thought disorder in which the patient displays an inability to change the topic or gives the same response to different questions. Thought insertion refers to the patient's idea that some thought content is being inserted directly into the patient's mind.

41. The answer is e. *(Ebert, p 107.)* Derealization is the subjective sense that the environment is strange or unreal, as if reality had been changed.

Perception is a physical sensation given a meaning or the integration of sensory stimuli to form an image or impression; in dulled perception, this capacity is diminished. Retardation of thought refers to the slowing of thought processes that may be seen in major depression. Response time to questions may be increased. Depersonalization refers to feeling that one is falling apart or not one's self, that one's self is unreal or detached.

42. The answer is b. *(Kaplan, p 282.)* Magical thinking is a form of thinking similar to that of preoperational phase children (Jean Piaget) in which thoughts and ideas are believed to have special powers (for example, to cause or stop outside events). In thought broadcasting, the patient senses that his or her thoughts are being stolen, are leaking out of the mind, or are being sent out to others across radio or television. Echolalia refers to the repetition of the examiner's words or phrases by the patient. Nihilism is the belief that oneself, others, or the world are either nonexistent or are coming to an end. An obsession is the ego-dystonic persistence of a thought or feeling that cannot be eliminated from consciousness voluntarily.

43. The answer is b. *(Goldman, 5/e, p 111.)* A compulsion is the need to act on an impulse (often an obsession) that is accompanied with anxiety if the impulse is resisted. Often the compulsion has no end in itself, other than to prevent something from occurring in the future. Catalepsy is the general term for an immobile position that is constantly maintained. Magical thinking is a form of thinking similar to that of preoperational phase children (Jean Piaget) in which thoughts and ideas are believed to have special powers (for example to cause or stop outside events). Anhedonia, which occurs frequently in major depressive disorders, is the lack of enjoyment or interest in outside pursuits or hobbies previously enjoyed. Folie à deux is a shared psychotic (delusional) belief held by two people.

44. The answer is d. *(Goldman, 5/e, p 112.)* Echopraxia is the mimicking of the examiner's body posture and movements by the patient. This can be seen in chronic schizophrenia. Folie à deux is a shared psychotic (delusional) belief held by two people. Dereistic thinking is a thought activity not concordant with logic or experience. Echolalia refers to the repetition of the examiner's words or phrases by the patient. Fugue is the taking on of a new identity with no memory of the old one. It often involves travel to a new environment.

45–47. The answers are 45-c, 46-e, 47-b. (*Goldman, 5/e, p 175.*) Axis I is the place to record all primary psychiatric disorders other than mental retardation or personality disorders, which are recorded on Axis II. Axis III is where medical conditions of all kinds, whether or not related to the primary psychiatric diagnosis, are recorded. Axis IV is the place to record stressors that are occurring in the patient's life—including social, legal, or financial situations. Axis V records the global assessment of functioning on a scale of 0 to 100.

Human Behavior: Theories of Personality and Development

Questions

DIRECTIONS: Each item below contains a question or incomplete statement followed by suggested responses. Select the **one best** response to each question.

48. A mother promptly responds to her infant's distress cries. Well attuned to his cues, she has no difficulty identifying the cause of the distress and she promptly attends to it. Shortly after, the infant smiles contentedly and the mother smiles back at him. Later in the day, the child spends 2 hours with a babysitter while the mother goes shopping. On his mother's return, he greets her with a great display of pleasure and outstretched arms. According to Bowlby's theory, which of the following best describes this child's behavior?

a. Oral phase
b. Infantile neurosis
c. Secure attachment
d. Imprinting
e. Easy temperament

49. A 10-year-old child is very interested in school and is proud of his athletic achievements. Peers are very important to him, but he also gets along with his parents. Under stress, he tends to become overly focused on details and slightly obsessive. At what stage is he, according to Sigmund Freud's theory of psychosexual development?

a. Concrete operational
b. Latency
c. Industry vs. inferiority
d. Object constancy
e. Separation-individuation

50. A 20-month-old boy loves running around and exploring the environment, but every few minutes he keeps returning to his mother to check on her and solicit a quick hug. Which of the following best describes this behavior, according to Margaret Mahler?
   a. Depressive position
   b. Secure attachment
   c. Insecure attachment
   d. Rapprochement
   e. Autonomy vs. shame and doubt

51. Margaret Mahler is best known for which of the following theories?
   a. Psychosocial development
   b. Psychosexual maturation
   c. Cognitive development
   d. Moral development
   e. Separation-individuation

52. Which of the following theorists primarily focused on the importance of early parental behavior such as mirroring, leading to the development of a cohesive and stable sense of self?
   a. Piaget
   b. Erikson
   c. Freud
   d. Klein
   e. Kohut

53. Piaget is best known for which of the following theories?
   a. Cognitive development
   b. Psychosexual development
   c. Psychosocial development
   d. Interpersonal development
   e. Attachment

Items 54–55

A 2-year-old child carries around an old, tattered blanket wherever he goes. When he is sad or upset, he calms himself down by hugging and stroking his blanket. He also needs it to settle down before sleep.

54. For this child, which of the following does this blanket represent?
a. Fetish
b. Obsession
c. Transitional object
d. Phallic substitute
e. Imaginary friend

55. Which of the following analysts introduced this concept?
a. Piaget
b. Klein
c. Kohut
d. Anna Freud
e. Winnicott

Items 56–57

A 3-year-old boy stands on one side of a large sculpture and is asked to describe what he sees. When asked to describe what a person on the other side of the sculpture sees, the child answers that the other person sees just what he does.

56. Which of the following best describes this kind of logic?
a. Autistic thinking
b. Concrete thinking
c. Egocentrism
d. Primary process
e. Object constancy

57. Which of the following theories uses the concept described above?
a. Psychosexual development
b. Moral development
c. Cognitive development
d. Social development
e. Autism

58. A 70-year-old woman has had three face-lifts and never leaves the house without makeup. She forbids her grandchildren to address her as "grandmother" and lies about her age. According to Erikson, which state of development is she having difficulty mastering?
a. Integrity vs. despair
b. Egocentric
c. Generativity vs. stagnation
d. Narcissistic
e. Pragmatic development

59. Which of the following statements is true about temperament?
a. It is biologically determined
b. It is unchangeable throughout life
c. It is always caused by poor parenting
d. Children with temperaments that are slow to warm up cannot be taught to be less fearful of change
e. It is a synonym for personality

60. A young woman with a history of childhood neglect feels suddenly worthless and devastated when her supervisor makes a mildly negative comment about her work performance. According to Heinz Kohut, her hypersensitivity to criticism is due to which of the following explanations?
a. An unresolved oedipal complex due to her parents' divorce when the woman was 4 years old
b. An inability to make stable commitments to others
c. A punitive superego due to harsh and critical parents
d. A fragmented sense of self due to the empathic failure of her parents
e. Autistic traits

61. Carl Jung, a psychoanalyst who once was a disciple of Freud, developed the concept of archetypes. Which of the following statements best defines an archetype?
a. Unconscious traits possessed by humans
b. Representational images and configurations with universal symbolic meanings
c. Feeling-tones—ideas that develop as a result of personal experience
d. A process by which people develop a unique sense of their own identity
e. An inner world of thoughts, intuitions, emotions, and sensations

62. A 23-year-old woman constantly goes to great lengths to avoid being criticized, even when this requires going against her own beliefs and wishes. Although she is good-looking and successful, she is tormented by doubts about her abilities and her physical appearance. According to Kohutian theory, which of the following explanations is the most likely to explain her behavior?

a. Overly harsh toilet training when she was 3 years old
b. Overindulgent parents who freely dispensed praise
c. A lack of self-esteem, which causes a constant need for validation
d. An overly punitive superego
e. A shy temperament

63. A 5-year-old boy is presented with two stories and asked which character has committed the worse infraction and should receive the more severe consequence. In the first story, a little boy breaks one cup when he climbs over the counter to reach a cake placed on top of the refrigerator. In the second story, a little girl breaks five cups and one plate by accident when she trips over the cat while she is helping her mother in the kitchen. Which of the following answers would most likely be chosen by this boy?

a. The little boy, because he broke the cup while he was trying to steal the cake, a forbidden act
b. The little girl, because she did more damage
c. The boy and the girl are equally guilty because both of them broke something and breaking things is wrong
d. The boy and girl have done nothing wrong, because they did not intend to break anything
e. The boy has committed the worse infraction, but only if he is found out

64. In psychoanalytic theory, which of the following statements is true about the superego?

a. It is totally unconscious
b. It is a defense mechanism
c. It functions to reduce guilt and shame
d. It includes the sexual and aggressive drives
e. It contains the ego ideal

65. A 20-month-old girl is admitted to a pediatric ward because she weighs only 15 lb. An extensive medical workup does not reveal any organic cause for the child's failure to thrive. The child is listless, apathetic, and does not smile. The parents rarely come to visit, and, when they do, they do not pick the child up and do not play or interact with her. Which of the following statements best explains this scenario?

a. Lack of adequate emotional nurturance causes depression and failure to thrive in infants
b. Neglected infants fail to thrive but do not have the intrapsychic structures necessary for experiencing depression
c. Infants reared in institutions are likely to become autistic
d. Neglected infants are at higher risk for developing schizophrenia
e. Environmental variables have little impact on the health of infants as long as enough food is provided

66. The effects of emotional deprivation on infants were extensively investigated by which psychoanalyst?

a. Melanie Klein
b. Erik Erikson
c. Otto Kernberg
d. Anna Freud
e. Renée Spitz

Items 67–68

A healthy 9-month-old girl, previously very friendly with everyone, now bursts into tears when she is approached by an unfamiliar adult.

67. Which of the following statements best describes this child's behavior?

a. Separation anxiety
b. Insecure attachment
c. Simple phobia
d. Depressive position
e. Stranger anxiety

68. Which of the following is true about this kind of behavior?
a. It is common in normal infants
b. It is always a symptom of insecure attachment
c. It is only present in children who will subsequently develop anxiety disorders
d. It is likely to persist if it is not adequately treated
e. It is a symptom of pervasive developmental disorder

69. A 25-month-old boy plays with a ball, which rolls under a couch. The boy promptly crawls under the couch to retrieve the ball. According to Piaget's theories of cognitive development, which thinking process best describes this child's behavior?
a. Object permanence
b. Basic trust
c. Initiative vs. guilt
d. Object constancy
e. Sensorimotor stage

70. According to Sigmund Freud, which of the following best describes primary processes?
a. Typically conscious
b. Nonlogical and primitive
c. Absent during dreaming
d. Characteristic of the neuroses
e. Rational and well organized

71. Harry Stack Sullivan's theory of personality development is characterized by which of the following emphases?
a. Psychosexual development
b. Genetic determinism
c. Infant-mother interaction
d. Interpersonal relations
e. Object relations

72. Erikson's developmental theories differ from Freud's in that Erikson placed greater emphasis on which of the following?
a. Cultural factors in development
b. Instinctual drives
c. Interpersonal relations
d. Psychosexual development
e. Object relations

73. A woman has a verbal altercation with her boss at work. She meekly accepts his harsh words. That night, she picks a fight with her husband. Which of the following defense mechanisms is being used by this woman?
a. Displacement
b. Acting out
c. Reaction formation
d. Projection
e. Sublimation

74. A 24-year-old woman lives with her mother, whom she intensely dislikes. She feels embarrassed by this, and compensates by hovering over her mother, attending to her every need. Which of the following defense mechanisms is being used by this woman?
a. Displacement
b. Acting out
c. Reaction formation
d. Rationalization
e. Sublimation

75. A writer of mystery novels who has never had legal problems jokes about his "dark side" and his hidden fantasies about leading an exciting life of crime. Which of the following defense mechanisms is being used by this man?
a. Anticipation
b. Sublimation
c. Identification with the aggressor
d. Introjection
e. Distortion

76. A 35-year-old man is being seen by his psychiatrist for depressed mood. The patient is irritated at his therapist for pushing him on several issues in the last session. The patient does not show up or call for his next session. Which of the following defense mechanisms is this patient displaying?

a. Introjection
b. Sublimation
c. Identification with the aggressor
d. Acting out
e. Intellectualization

77. A 45-year-old man crashes his car into another vehicle by accident. He feels extremely guilty and, in order to avoid these feelings of self-reproach, he explains in meticulous detail to anyone listening all of the steps leading up to his accident. Which of the following defense mechanisms is this patient displaying?

a. Sublimation
b. Repression
c. Intellectualization
d. Acting out
e. Rationalization

Psychiatry

DIRECTIONS: Each group of questions below consists of lettered options followed by a set of numbered items. For each numbered item, select the **one** lettered option with which it is **most** closely associated. Each lettered option may be used once, more than once, or not at all.

Items 78–80

Match the following situations with the correct concept.
a. Core identity
b. Gender role
c. Gender identity
d. Sexual identity
e. Sexual drive

78. A 3-year-old both knows that he is a male "like Daddy" and becomes upset if someone mistakes him for a little girl. **(CHOOSE 1 CONCEPT)**

79. A 14-year-old girl spends a great deal of time putting on makeup and styling her hair. She babysits after school and likes to cook. She considers heavy yard work a job more suited to her brother. **(CHOOSE 1 CONCEPT)**

80. A 23-year-old man enjoys the company of women and is sexually aroused by them. **(CHOOSE 1 CONCEPT)**

Items 81–82

Match the patient's symptoms with the correct diagnosis.
a. Punishment dream
b. Displacement
c. Secondary revision
d. Preconscious
e. Condensation

81. A 24-year-old woman tells her psychiatrist that she had a dream in which her mother, with a suit and tie on, just like the psychiatrist usually wears, told her to take out the garbage, just like her father used to tell her. Which of the terms above best describes the details of this dream? **(CHOOSE 1 DIAGNOSIS)**

82. A 40-year-old man reports to his psychiatrist that he had a dream in which he murdered his aunt, a woman with whom the patient had little contact. The psychiatrist noted that the patient's unconscious had probably substituted the aunt for the mother in the dream, since there was much evidence that the patient was very angry with her. Which of the terms above best describes what the psychiatrist thinks occurred in this dream? **(CHOOSE 1 DIAGNOSIS)**

83. A 42-year-old man is seen in the emergency room with the chief complaint of suicidal ideation. After he is hospitalized, his doctor discovers that he is faking his psychiatric symptoms in order to escape an outstanding warrant for his arrest. Which of the following terms best describes this patient's behavior?
a. Primary gain
b. Secondary gain
c. Wish fulfillment
d. Acting out
e. Psychic determinism

Items 84–87

Match the description of each psychoanalytic theory with the correct theorist.
a. Sigmund Freud
b. John Bowlby
c. Heinz Kohut
d. Melanie Klein
e. Erik Erikson
f. Jean Piaget

84. Which of these psychoanalytic theorists wrote about signal anxiety as a result of conflicts between the id, ego, and superego? **(CHOOSE 1 THEORIST)**

85. Which of the psychoanalytic theorists wrote about the epigenetic principle that development occurs in sequential, clearly defined stages? **(CHOOSE 1 THEORIST)**

86. Which of the psychoanalytic theorists wrote about anxiety caused by the patient's disruption of attachment to parents in infancy? **(CHOOSE 1 THEORIST)**

87. Which of the psychoanalytic theorists wrote about the four major stages (sensorimotor, preoperational thought, concrete operations, and formal operations) that a child must pass through leading to the capacity for adult thought? **(CHOOSE 1 THEORIST)**

Items 88–89

88. The parents of a 2-year-old child come to see the child's pediatrician because their once happy-go-lucky infant has become oppositional and obstinate. According to Freudian theory, which of the following developmental stages is this child in?

a. Oral
b. Anal
c. Phallic
d. Oedipal
e. Latency

89. A 5-year-old girl loves her father's attention and becomes irritated with her mother when her mother kisses her father. The child tells her father she wants to marry him when she grows up. According to Freudian theory, which of the following developmental stages is this child in?

a. Oral
b. Anal
c. Phallic
d. Oedipal
e. Latency

90. Which of Freud's theories deals with a model of the mind divided into three regions—the conscious, unconscious, and preconscious?

a. Parapraxes
b. Infantile sexuality
c. Structural
d. Topographic
e. Primary process

Items 91–93

91. A young man in a conflicted relationship with a woman who reminds him of his domineering mother dreams that he is having tea with a woman who has his fiancee's features but his mother's eyes and hair color. In the dream, the young man realizes with horror that he is paralyzed from the waist down. He tries to communicate his distress to his fiancee, but she is oblivious and continues talking about buying new furniture. With an enormous effort, the young man manages to stand up, and at that moment the woman in this dream starts floating in the air as a balloon and disappears. According to Freud's theories, the dream may represent an insight into the fact that his fiancee has emotionally paralyzed the dreamer, as his mother had done before her. Which of the following elements of a dream does this insight represent?
a. Manifest content of the dream
b. Latent content of the dream
c. Dream work
d. Punishment dream
e. Defense mechanism

92. Which of the following represents the process that transforms the raw unconscious wishes and impulses of the dreamer into images more acceptable to the superego?
a. Manifest content of the dream
b. Latent content of the dream
c. Dream work
d. Punishment dream
e. Defense mechanism

93. The illogical, bizarre, and incoherent images that often make up dreams are an example of what type of thinking?
a. Primary process
b. Dream anxiety
c. Manifest content
d. Secondary process
e. Secondary revision

Human Behavior: Theories of Personality and Development

Answers

48. The answer is c. *(Ebert, p 11.)* John Bowlby, a psychiatrist who published most of his work between 1970 and 1990, is known for his work on infant attachment. He theorized that infants are predisposed from birth to form attachments with their primary caregivers and that the quality of the attachment depends on their caregivers' response to them. When the caregiver is attentive and responsive to the infant's physical and emotional needs, secure attachment is the norm. Insecure attachment occurs when the caregiver is unresponsive, neglectful, or inconsistent. The quality of attachment has been empirically studied through the strange situation procedure, which focuses on the infant's reaction when he or she is reunited with the parent after a brief separation. Children with secure attachment greet their parents with relatively unequivocal pleasure (like the child in this vignette). Children with insecure attachment manifest a variety of deviant behaviors, stemming from their lack of confidence that the parent will be helpful and available. Behaviors associated with insecure attachment include avoiding or ignoring the parent; anger and aggression; extreme passivity; clingy, whiny behavior; or a combination of all these.

Basic trust also describes a stage of development characterized by the security that caregivers will be helpful and available on the basis of the quality of the child's previous interactions. This phase is the first of Erikson's eight psychosocial developmental stages and does not belong to Bowlby's theories. The oral phase is the first of the five psychosexual developmental stages theorized by Freud. The term infantile neurosis describes, in Freudian psychoanalytic theory of development, the appearance of regressive behaviors and fears during the oedipal period as an attempt to withdraw from the conflicts caused by the intensity of the oedipal longing for the parent of the opposite sex. Imprinting refers to an instinctual attachment system in which certain stimuli are capable of eliciting innate behavior patterns during the first few hours of an animal's behavioral development, allowing the offspring to become attached to its mother very early in a critical period of development. Temperament refers to an inherited set of personality traits such as adaptability, intensity of reaction, threshold of responsiveness, and so forth. A difficult temperament may affect attachment, because it makes parenting more frustrating and can interfere with the parent's ability to relate to the child positively.

49. The answer is b. *(Kaplan, 8/e, p 216.)* According to Freud's psychosexual developmental theory, children between the age of 5 and 12 or 13 enter into a stage where sexual drives become secondary (hence the term latency) while other developmental tasks, such as peer relations and school achievements, become more important. Children at this stage have a strong sense of right and wrong and like to play by the rules. Usually there is a tendency toward orderliness, attention to details, and collecting things. Under stress, these traits may become exaggerated. The stormy parent-child relationship that characterizes adolescence is yet to come. Industry vs. inferiority and the concrete operational stage apply to the same age period, respectively, in Erikson's psychosocial developmental theory and Piaget's theory of cognitive development. Separation and individuation and object constancy refer to two stages of infant development according to Margaret Mahler's theory.

50. The answer is d. *(Kaplan, 8/e, p 36.)* Margaret Mahler made her contributions to the psychoanalytic movement called ego psychology through her theories on early infantile development. On the basis of her observations of normal and pathological mother-child interactions, Mahler identified three developmental phases of infant development. The autistic phase occurs during the first 2 months of life, when the child spends a good part of his or her day asleep and has little interest in interpersonal relationships. From 2 to 6 months, the child enters symbiosis, a stage characterized by psychological fusion or lack of differentiation between mother and child. Margaret Mahler is best known, however, for her research on the third phase, called separation-individuation. During this phase, which occurs between 6 and 36 months, the child develops a concept of him- or herself as different and separated from the mother. During the same period, the infant gradually develops an internal, stable representation (introjection) of the mother, which includes both her positive and negative aspects. The separation-individuation phase is divided into four subphases: differentiation, between 6 and 10 months, refers to the child's initial awareness that the mother is a separate person; practicing, between 10 and 16 months, is characterized by the child's enthusiastic exploration of the environment, thanks to his or her newly acquired mobility; rapprochement, between 16 and 24 months, refers to a period characterized by a need to know where the mother is and frequent "refueling," triggered by the child's new awareness that independence also makes him or her vulnerable; the fourth subphase, object constancy, takes place during the third year of life and refers to the integration of the good and bad aspects of both the internalized images of the mother and the child's self. According to ego psychology theory, object constancy is necessary for the later development of stable and mature interpersonal relationships.

In Melanie Klein's theory of infantile psychological development, the depressive position refers to the period during which the infant realizes that the "bad mother" who frustrates the child's wishes and the "good mother" who nurtures him or her are the same person and the child worries that rage at the "bad mother" may also destroy the good. Autonomy vs. shame and doubt is one of the eight stages of psychosocial development described by Erikson and corresponds in age to the period of Mahler's separation-individuation.

51. The answer is e. (*Kaplan, 8/e, p 36.*) Margaret Mahler is best known for her theory of separation-individuation. (See answer 50 for more detail on her theories.) Erik Erikson is known for his theory of psychosocial development throughout the life cycle. Freud's theories relate to the child's psychosexual development and to the role unconscious conflicts play in psychopathology. Piaget is known for his work on cognitive development. Lawrence Kohlberg integrated Piaget's concepts and described three major levels of morality: preconventional, in which punishment and obedience to the parent are the determining factors; morality of conventional role-conformity, in which children try to conform to gain approval and to maintain good relationships with others; and morality of self-accepted moral principles, in which children voluntarily comply with rules on the basis of a concept of ethical principles.

52. The answer is e. (*Kaplan, 8/e, p 228.*) Heinz Kohut is one of the founders of one of the three modern psychoanalytic schools, Self-Psychology. He theorized that in order to develop a coherent, stable, and resilient sense of self, the child needs positive, empathic, and consistent responses from his or her caretakers. The need for positive and validating responses from the environment is not limited to infancy or childhood, since even adults need a certain amount of positive feedback from others to maintain positive self-esteem. Individuals whose sense of self remains fragile and unstable due to faulty early parenting need constant and excessive reassurance from others and become emotionally and behaviorally dysfunctional under stress. Freud's theories relate to the child's psychosexual development and to the role unconscious conflicts play in psychopathology. Erik Erikson is known for his theory of psychosocial development throughout the life cycle. Melanie Klein is a proponent of the object relations school of psychoanalysis and wrote extensively on early stages of infant-mother interaction. Piaget is known for his work on cognitive development.

53. The answer is a. *(Kaplan, 8/e, p 141.)* Jean Piaget, a Swiss psychologist, made extensive empirical observations of the way children reason and make sense of their environment at various ages. His theory of the development of cognitive thinking in children encompasses four stages: sensorimotor (18 to 24 months), preoperational (2 through 5 to 7 years), concrete operational (6 to 11 years), and formal operational (11 years to adulthood). Each stage is characterized by specific ways of approaching and processing information.

54. The answer is c. *(Goldman, 5/e, p 35.)* D. W. Winnicott, a British pediatrician with a keen interest in psychoanalysis, focused his attention on the early mother-child relationship. In his view, the child is able to develop a separate and stable identity only if the child's needs are met by his or her mother's empathic anticipation. Winnicott calls the positive environment so created by the mother the *holding environment*. According to Winnicott, mothers do not have to be perfect in order to fulfill their roles, but they have to be good enough to provide the infant with a sufficient amount of comfort and constancy. Winnicott also coined the term *transitional object*, usually a toy or a blanket, that represents a comforting substitute for the primary caregiver. Thanks to a transitional object, the child can tolerate separation from the mother without excessive anxiety.

55. The answer is e. *(Goldman, 5/e, p 35.)* D. W. Winnicott, a British pediatrician with a keen interest in psychoanalysis, focused his attention on the early mother-child relationship. (See answer 54 for more detail on Winnicott's theories.)

56–57. The answers are 56-c, 57-c. *(Goldman, 5/e, p 34.)* Egocentrism refers to young children's inability to see things from another point of view. Egocentrism is described by Jean Piaget as part of the preoperational stage of cognitive development, which occurs between 2 and 5 to 7 years of age.

58. The answer is a. *(Kaplan, 8/e, p 235.)* Erik Erikson's theory of psychosocial development centers around eight stages of ego development that take place during the life cycle. Each stage represents a turning point in which physical, cognitive, social, and emotional changes trigger an internal crisis whose resolution results either in psychological growth or regression. Integrity vs. despair is the last of the Eriksonian stages and takes place between age 60 and death. If this stage is successfully mastered, the individual arrives at a peaceful acceptance of his or her mortality without losing interest in life. The woman in the question, with her futile attempts to deny the passage of time, clearly has difficulties in this developmental stage. The other developmental stages in Erikson's theory are as follows: (1) trust vs. mistrust, which occurs between birth and 18 months of age. During this period, if the infant's needs are promptly and empathically met, the infant learns to see the world as a benign and nurturing place. (2) Autonomy vs. shame and doubt, which occurs between 18 months and 3 years and corresponds to Freud's anal stage and Mahler's separation-individuation stage. During this period, if allowed to experiment with his or her new motility and curiosity about the environment, and if at the same time he or she is provided enough nurturance, the child acquires a healthy self-esteem and sense of autonomy. (3) Initiative vs. guilt, which occurs between 3 and 5 years of age, when the child expands his or her explorations of the outside world and has omnipotent fantasies about his or her own powers. During this stage, in a good psychosocial environment, the child develops a capacity of self-reflection, manifested by feeling guilty when rules are broken, without losing enthusiasm for independent exploration. (4) Industry vs. inferiority, which occurs between 5 and 13 years of age, is equivalent to Freud's period of latency. The child's psychological growth depends on his or her opportunity to learn new skills and to take pride in accomplishments. (5) identity vs. role confusion, which occurs during adolescence, between approximately 13 and 21 years. If this stage is mastered successfully, the young individual enters adulthood with a solid sense of identity, knowing his or her role in society. (6) Intimacy vs. isolation, which refers to the adult developmental task of learning to make and honor commitments to other people and to ideas. (7) Generativity vs. stagnation, which occurs between 40 and 60 years of age. According to Erikson, the focus of the individual starts shifting from personal accomplishments and needs to a concern for the rest of society and the nurturing of the next generation. (8) Integrity vs. despair, which occurs from approximately age 60 to death. The main developmental task is accepting life as it is, without desire to change the past or change others. When this stage is mastered, the individual acquires the wisdom necessary to face the inevitability of death with equanimity and without dread.

59. The answer is a. *(Kaplan, 8/e, p 35.)* Temperament refers to an inherited set of traits that are present at birth and are rather stable during the first years of life, although they can often be modified by interpersonal and other experiences later on. Three temperamental styles are described, on the basis of variations in several categories such as rhythmicity, adaptability, intensity of reaction, quality of mood, attention span, and so forth. Children with an easy temperament—approximately 40% of the population—are adaptable to changes, have regular feeding and sleeping rhythms, have a predominantly pleasant mood, and have responses of mild or moderate intensity. Children with a difficult temperament, on the contrary, adapt slowly to change, have irregular biological rhythms, and have frequent high-intensity negative emotional displays. Children with a slow-to-warm-up temperament, usually labeled as "shy," tend to withdraw from new experiences and have negative emotional responses with low intensity. Although quality of parenting does not cause a specific temperament, temperament can affect parenting styles. For example, children with difficult temperaments are more likely to elicit negative responses and, in extreme cases, abusive behaviors from caregivers.

60. The answer is d. *(Ebert, p 46.)* According to Kohut, empathic validation from caregivers is essential for the development of an integrated sense of self. People who have been neglected or abused or have received suboptimal parenting grow up with a very fragile sense of self and an easily shaken self-esteem. These individuals, like the woman in the question, cannot maintain a positive image of themselves when exposed to criticism or rejection and experience a devastating sense of worthlessness and fragmentation.

61. The answer is b. *(Kaplan, 8/e, p 227.)* Carl Jung, a contemporary and disciple of Freud, who later moved away from classical Freudian psychoanalytic theory, defined the "shadow" as a part of the unconscious personality that contains all the traits and qualities that are unacceptable to an individual. For example, for a generous person, avarice is a shadow quality. On the contrary, for a person that takes pride in frugality, generosity is part of the shadow. Archetypes, also part of Jungian psychology, are universal, symbolic images that recur in dreams and are part of the "collective unconscious." The animus, according to Jung, contains the masculine elements of a woman's personality, while the anima represents the female traits of a man's personality.

62. The answer is c. *(Ebert, p 46.)* According to Kohut's theories, individuals who require other people's constant validation to maintain a marginal self-esteem have suffered a "narcissistic injury" during childhood due to parental neglect or lack of empathy.

63. The answer is b. *(Kaplan, 8/e, pp 34, 45.)* According to the theories of moral development of Piaget and Kohlberg, for children between 4 and 7 years of age, the consequence of an action determines its intrinsic moral value independently from the intention and circumstances. At this age, children see rules as permanent and unchangeable, and punishment is dispensed by figures of authority without a possibility of appeal. Older children (7 to 14) make moral judgments taking into account the intent of the doer and the situational circumstances.

64. The answer is e. *(Kaplan, 8/e, p 217.)* In his structural theory of the mind, Freud divided the psychic apparatus into three agencies: the id, which contains the instinctual drives; the ego, whose function is to find an equilibrium between gratification of the instinctual drives and the rules of society (and the demands of the superego); and the superego, the agency that contains the internalized parental and societal rules and dictates to the ego what is not to be done. The ego ideal, a component of the superego, is the internal standard of what one should be to be approved all the time by

Human Behavior: Theories of Personality and Development Answers

society and internalized parental figures. Shame is a consequence of not living up to one's ego ideal, while guilt is the consequence of transgressing the superego's prohibitions. The superego, as well as the ego, have both conscious and unconscious components.

65. The answer is a. (*Ebert, p 537.*) Although the relationships between emotional deprivation and failure to thrive are complex, the fact that children who are emotionally deprived do not grow well, even when an adequate amount of food is available, is well proven. Renée Spitz studied institutionalized children and demonstrated that, due to lack of adequate nurturing, they become apathetic, withdrawn, and less interested in feeding, which in turn causes failure to thrive and, in extreme cases, death. Spitz called this syndrome *anaclitic depression.* Schizophrenia and autism have not been associated with emotional deprivation in infancy.

66. The answer is e. (*Kaplan, 8/e, p 36.*) Renée Spitz studied institutionalized children and demonstrated that, due to lack of adequate nurturing, they become apathetic, withdrawn, and less interested in feeding, which in turn causes failure to thrive and, in extreme cases, death. Spitz called this syndrome *anaclitic depression.*

67–68. The answers are 67-e, 68-a. (*Kaplan, 8/e, p 36.*) The term *stranger anxiety* refers to manifestations of discomfort and distress on the part of the infant when he or she is approached by a stranger. Although it does not necessarily appear every time the child meets a stranger, and although some children seem to be more prone than others to such reactions, stranger anxiety is considered a normal, transient phenomenon. It manifests at about 8 months of age, when the child starts differentiating between familiar and unfamiliar adults.

69. The answer is a. (*Kaplan, 8/e, p 141.*) According to Piaget, object permanence is the recognition that an object continues to exist even if it cannot be perceived. Object permanence is reached during the preoperational stage of cognitive development, which extends from 2 to 6 years of age. The child in the question understands that, even if he cannot see the ball anymore, the toy still exists under the couch. A younger child who has not yet reached the stage of object permanence would consider the ball as lost forever. Object permanence is often confused with object constancy, a psychoanalytic concept referring to children's ability to maintain stable, realistic internalized constructs of their caretakers and themselves. Object constancy is a fundamental concept in ego psychology and Self-Psychology.

70. The answer is b. *(Kaplan, 8/e, p 217.)* Primary process thinking is primitive, nonlogical, and timeless. Primary processes characterize the operational style of the id and are manifested in dreams. According to Freud's theory, condensation, displacement, and symbolic representation are forms of primary processes.

71. The answer is d. *(Kaplan, 8/e, p 16.)* Harry Stack Sullivan's theory of personality development emphasizes the central importance of interpersonal relationships. He believed that the interpersonal relationships of the first 5 years of life were crucial, although not immutable, in shaping personality. He thought that personality continues to develop and change throughout adolescence and into adulthood and that, in therapy, the opportunity for change derives from an active interaction between patient and therapist.

72. The answer is a. *(Kaplan, 8/e, p 234.)* Erikson's work concentrated on the effects of social, cultural, and psychological factors in development. Although Erikson acknowledged the important role of sexuality, it was less central to his theory. The concepts of instinctual drives and psychosexual development are essential parts of Freud's theories. Object relations, which refers not to interpersonal relationships but to the interactions of internalized constructs of external relationships, is the central idea in object relation psychology.

73. The answer is a. *(Goldman, 5/e, p 6.)* In Freudian psychoanalytic theory, defense mechanisms represent the ego's attempts to mediate between the pressure of the instinctual drives, emerging from the id, and the restrictions imposed by societal rules through the superego. Freud classified defense mechanisms as narcissistic (or primitive, including denial, projection, and distortion), immature (acting out, introjection, passive-aggressive behavior, somatization, and several others), neurotic (displacement, externalization, intellectualization, rationalization, inhibition, reaction formation, and repression), and mature (sublimation, altruism, asceticism, anticipation, suppression, and humor). Primitive and immature defenses are the norm during childhood and infancy and persist in pathological states. Mature defenses are considered more adaptive than immature and neurotic defenses.

In displacement, an unacceptable impulse or emotion is shifted from one object to another. This permits the release of the impulse or emotion onto someone or something that is less unacceptable or dangerous. In this case, although the woman is angry at her boss, it is too dangerous to release this anger at him (she might be fired). She waits until she gets home and displaces this anger onto her husband. Projection is a defense mechanism in which the patient reacts to an inner unacceptable impulse as if it were outside the self.

74. The answer is c. *(Goldman, 5/e, p 6.)* In reaction formation, an unacceptable unconscious impulse is transformed into its opposite. Rationalization refers to offering a rational explanation to justify actions or impulses that would otherwise be regarded as unacceptable.

75. The answer is b. *(Goldman, 5/e, p 5.)* Through sublimation, satisfaction of an objectionable impulse is obtained by using socially acceptable means. The writer in the question derives a vicarious satisfaction of his antisocial impulses through the criminal activities of the characters of his stories. Identification refers to the incorporation of another person's qualities into one's ego system. Introjection refers to the internalization of the qualities of an object. For example, through the introjection of a loved object, the painful awareness of separateness or the threat of loss may be avoided. Distortion refers to the gross reshaping of external reality to suit inner needs. Distortions include hallucinations and delusions.

76. The answer is d. *(Goldman, 5/e, p 6.)* Acting out means the avoidance of personally unacceptable feelings by behaving in a socially inappropriate manner that is often attention-seeking as well. Acting out implies the expression of an impulse through action to avoid experiencing the accompanying effect at a conscious level. Intellectualization is the excessive use of intellectual processes to avoid affective expression or experience.

77. The answer is c. *(Goldman, 5/e, p 6.)* Intellectualization is the excessive use of intellectual processes to avoid affective expression or experience. In this case, the man avoids his guilty feelings through the meticulous explanation, over and over, of the events leading up to his car accident. Through sublimation, satisfaction of an objectionable impulse is obtained by using socially acceptable means. Repression refers to the expelling or withholding from consciousness an idea or feeling. Acting out implies the expression of an impulse through action to avoid experiencing the accompanying effect at a conscious level. Rationalization is the process of offering rational explanations in an attempt to justify attitudes, beliefs, or behavior that may otherwise be unacceptable.

78–80. The answers are 78-c, 79-b, 80-d. *(Goldman, 5/e, p 367.)* Gender identity, a deep-rooted awareness of being either male or female, seems to depend in great part on the way the individual is reared, as a boy or a girl. Once established, usually by age 2 or 3, it is extremely resistant to change. In gender identity disorders, individuals identify strongly with the opposite sex and dislike their own sexual characteristics. Gender role refers to the many behaviors, such as wearing dresses and makeup vs. wearing pants and neckties, that identify an individual as male or female. It is not as unchangeable as gender identity and usually tends to fluctuate during the life course due to changes in beliefs, attitudes, and social mores (for example, smoking was considered a behavior unfit for women, but this later changed). Sexual identity refers to a subjective experience of an individual's sexual orientation and includes the awareness of what the individual considers sexually desirable.

81–82. The answers are 81-e, 82-b. *(Kaplan, 8/e, p 211.)* Condensation refers to the fact that several unconscious impulses, wishes, or feelings can be combined and attached to one manifest dream image. Composite characters often occur in dreams. Punishment dreams are dreams in which dreamers experience punishment. Freud understood them as reflective of the compromise between the repressed wish and the repressing agency or conscience. Displacement occurs in dreams to divert the energy associated with an object to a more suitable substitute (one that is more acceptable to the dreamer's ego). Secondary revision is the process by which the more mature and reasonable aspects of the ego work to organize primitive aspects of dreams into a more coherent form. The preconscious is one of the three regions of the mind (the other two are the conscious and the unconscious) described in Freud's topographical model.

Human Behavior: Theories of Personality and Development   *Answers*   55

83. The answer is b. *(Ebert, p 379.)* Primary gain refers to the relief of tension and conflict produced by the development of symptoms. In addition to the internal reduction of distress, the symptoms may gratify wishes or impulses (secondary gain). Examples of secondary gain include an increase in attention and sympathy, relief from burdensome obligations, and monetary compensation. Wish fulfillment is the term used by Freud to describe one of the goals of dreams. Acting out implies the expression of an impulse through action to avoid experiencing the accompanying effect at a conscious level. Freud's theory of psychic determinism refers to his belief that all mental events are in some way connected.

84–87. The answers are 84-a, 85-e, 86-b, 87-f. *(Kaplan, 8/e, pp 140, 145, 217, 234.)* In Freudian psychoanalytic theory, signal anxiety represents an autonomous function of the ego that activates unconscious defenses when impulses unacceptable to the superego threaten to emerge into consciousness. John Bowlby's work focused on infant attachment. In Bowlby's view, anxiety follows an insecure attachment caused by inconsistent or neglectful parenting. Heinz Kohut's theories hold that empathic, validating, and consistent responses from the parents or other primary caregivers are essential in the development of a cohesive and resilient self-concept. In Kohut's theories, developmental intrapsychic deficits caused by early empathic failures are involved in the development of personality disorders and manifest themselves through a multitude of emotional and behavioral dysfunctions, including anxiety. Melanie Klein evolved a theory of internal object relations that was intimately linked to drives. She viewed projection and introjection as the primary defensive operations in the first months of life. Erik Erikson formulated a theory of human development that covers the entire span of the life cycle, from infancy and childhood through old age and senescence. (See answer 58 for a further discussion of Erikson's theories.) Jean Piaget was interested in cognitive development and described four major stages leading to the capacity for adult thought (sensorimotor, preoperational thought, concrete operations, formal operations).

88–89. The answers are 88-b, 89-d. *(Kaplan, 8/e, pp 214, 215.)* According to Freud's theory of psychosexual development, the child goes through six stages between birth and adolescence: oral, anal, phallic, oedipal, latency, and genital. In each stage, pleasure (not necessarily sexual) is derived from specific areas of the body. Each stage is associated with specific drives, conflicts, and defenses.

In the first 18 months of life, infants go through the oral stage, during which oral sensations (feeding, sucking, biting, etc.) represent the main gratification. According to Freud, excessive gratification or deprivation during this stage can cause an "oral fixation." Individuals with an oral character are dependent and require that others fulfill their needs. In the anal stage, between 18 and 36 months of age, the child is much more independent and active than during the previous stage. Erotic stimulation of the anal mucosa through the excretion or retention of feces is the main source of pleasure. Battles over toilet training are common in the attempts to achieve autonomy from the parents. If toilet training is too harsh or inconsistent, "anal traits" may persist as personality traits later in life. Stubbornness, obstinacy, and frugality are common traits of the "anal individual," usually seen in obsessive-compulsive personalities. The phallic stage, which starts at age 3, is characterized by a concentration of erotic pleasure in the penis and the clitoris areas. During the phallic stage, the child starts looking outside himself or herself for an erotic object, thus heralding the advent of the oedipal stage. Freud theorized that between the ages of 3 and 5, the male child, like Oedipus in Greek mythology, falls in love with the mother and perceives the father as a murderous rival. Resolution of the oedipal stage leads to the boy's identification with the father and the abandonment of the erotic wishes for the mother, which are later transferred to other women. During the oedipal stage, girls experience an equivalent attraction for their fathers and perceive their mothers as rivals. How girls resolve their oedipal conflicts and come to identify with their mothers is less clearly explained. During latency, between 5 and 11 to 13 years of age, the sexual drive is relatively quiescent and the child becomes focused on learning new skills and social interactions with peers. The genital stage begins with puberty and ends with young adulthood and is characterized by a reintensification of sexual drives. The key developmental tasks associated with this stage are mastery over instinctual drives, separation from parents, and the establishment of a genital sexuality with an appropriate partner.

90. The answer is d. *(Kaplan, 8/e, p 211.)* The topographic model of the mind divides the mind into three regions: the conscious (that part of the mind in which perceptions coming from the outside world or from within the body or mind are brought into awareness), the preconscious (those mental events, processes, and contents capable of being brought into conscious awareness by the act of focusing attention), and the unconscious (mental contents and processes kept from conscious awareness through the force of censorship or repression). Parapraxes are unwitting slips of the tongue that reveal the unconscious at work. Infantile sexuality is a Freudian developmental theory of childhood sexuality that delineates the vicissitudes of erotic activity from birth through puberty. The structural theory of the mind describes the three psychic apparatuses—the ego, the id, and the superego—all distinguished by their different functions. Primary process refers to thinking that is dereistic, illogical, or magical; it is normally found in dreams and abnormally in psychosis.

91–93. The answers are 91-b, 92-c, 93-a. *(Kaplan, 8/e, pp 210, 211.)* One of Freud's main accomplishments was his observation that dreams are meaningful and that they provide valuable information about the dreamer's unconscious, although their meaning is often hidden or disguised. According to Freud's theory, each dream has a manifest content, which refers to images and sensations recalled by the dreamer, and a hidden latent content, represented by impulses, ideas, and feelings unacceptable to the conscious mind. Dream work is the process through which the latent content of the dream is transformed into the more acceptable manifest content. To disguise the latent content, the mind combines different concepts or feelings into one single image (condensation), uses neutral or innocent images to represent highly charged ideas or impulses (symbolic representation), and diverts the feeling or the energy associated with one object to another more acceptable to the dreamer's superego (displacement). Condensation, displacement, and symbolic representation are primary processes and can make the manifest content of the dream quite bizarre. Secondary revision, a process guided by the ego, intervenes at the end of the dream work to make the manifest content more rational and acceptable to the dreamer.

Human Behavior: Biologic and Related Sciences

Questions

DIRECTIONS: Each item below contains a question or incomplete statement followed by suggested responses. Select the **one best** response to each question.

94. A young man is often the object of his friends' jokes because he drops to the floor whenever he is having a good laugh. Which of the following findings is this man suffering from?

a. Cataplexy
b. Narcolepsy
c. Hysteria
d. Drop seizures
e. Histrionic personality

95. A young woman with a history of severe childhood abuse cuts or burns herself when she feels angry or anxious. She claims that hurting herself calms her and causes no pain. Self-injury can have this effect because it triggers the release of which of the following substances?

a. ACTH
b. Endorphins
c. Serotonin
d. Substance P
e. Arachidonic acid

96. Benzodiazepines, barbiturates, and many anticonvulsants exert their influence through which of the following types of receptors?

a. Muscarinic
b. Dopaminergic
c. Glutamic
d. Adrenergic
e. γ-aminobutyric acid (GABA)-ergic

97. The observation that levodopa (a drug used to treat Parkinson's disease) can cause mania and psychosis in some patients supports which neurochemical hypothesis?
a. Norepinephrine
b. Dopamine
c. Glycine
d. Serotonin
e. Glutamine

98. Seasonal circadian rhythm has been implicated in the etiology of which of the following psychopathologies?
a. Major depression
b. Schizophrenia
c. Borderline personality disorder
d. Panic disorder
e. Obsessive-compulsive disorder

99. A 46-year-old man is being monitored in a sleep study lab. After he has been asleep for 90 min, his EEG shows low-voltage, random fast activity with sawtooth waves. When awoken during this period, the patient reports he was dreaming. Which of the following sleep stages was this patient in when awakened?
a. Alpha waves
b. Theta waves
c. Sleep spindles
d. Delta waves
e. REM

100. After being struck on the head by a four-by-four, a previously serious and dependable construction worker starts making inappropriate sexual remarks to his co-workers, is easily distracted, and loses his temper over minor provocations. What part of his brain has been damaged?
a. Occipital lobe
b. Temporal lobe
c. Limbic system
d. Basal ganglion
e. Frontal lobe

101. A little girl who was underweight and hypotonic in infancy is obsessed with food, eats compulsively, and, at age 4, is already grossly overweight. She is argumentative, oppositional, and rigid. She has a narrow face, almond-shaped eyes, and a small mouth. Which of the following is the most likely diagnosis?

a. Down syndrome
b. Fragile X syndrome
c. Fetal alcohol syndrome
d. Hypothyroidism
e. Prader-Willi syndrome

102. A 36-year-old moderately retarded man with a long head, large ears, and hyperextensible joints is very shy and starts rocking and flapping his hands when he is upset. His disorder, the second most common single cause of mental retardation, is which of the following?

a. Down syndrome
b. Hurler's syndrome
c. Williams' syndrome
d. Fragile X syndrome
e. Rett's disorder

103. Monoamine oxidase inhibitors (MAOIs) exert their influence primarily by which of the following mechanisms?

a. Increasing GABA production
b. Blocking inactivation of biogenic amines
c. Decreasing norepinephrine
d. Decreasing serotonin
e. Increasing endorphin production

104. A 36-year-old woman is being evaluated in the sleep lab. She is noted to have a decreased latency of REM. Which of the following disorders is this woman most likely to be suffering from?

a. Schizophrenia
b. Major depression
c. Panic disorder
d. Obsessive-compulsive disorder
e. Posttraumatic stress disorder

105. A 17-year-old boy is brought to the emergency room by his friends after he "took a few pills" at a party and developed physical symptoms including his neck twisting to one side, his eyes rolling upward, and his tongue hanging out of his mouth. The patient responds immediately to 50 mg of diphenhydramine intramuscularly with the resolution of all physical symptoms. Which of the following substances is most likely to have caused the symptoms?
a. Methamphetamine
b. Meperidine
c. Alprazolam
d. Methylphenidate
e. Haloperidol

106. A 52-year-old housewife has gained weight although she has no increased appetite. She feels tired all the time and does not seem to care about anything anymore. She complains of being cold all the time. On exam, she appears depressed, her hair is dry and brittle, and her face is puffy. Which of the following laboratory findings is she likely to have?
a. Elevated ACTH
b. Low cortisol level
c. Elevated TSH
d. Low calcium level
e. Elevated FSH

107. A 32-year-old woman is brought to the emergency room after she complained of chest pain. She is noted to be hypervigilant and anxious, with a pulse of 120/min and a BP of 140/97. She has widely dilated pupils. Her toxicology screen is positive. Which of the following drugs is most likely the one found?
a. Cocaine
b. Ritalin
c. Heroin
d. PCP
e. LSD

108. The cell bodies of serotonin-releasing neurons are located in which area of the brain?

a. Raphe nuclei
b. Basal ganglia
c. Limbic system
d. Substantia nigra
e. Amygdaloid body

109. A 65-year-old woman with a history of chronic alcohol abuse cheerfully greets the resident doctor of her nursing home, whom she has met many times before, and calls him "my dear friend Jack." The physician explains who he is and tells the patient his name. Two minutes later, when he asks the patient if she knows who he is, she answers with a smile: "Of course, you are my cousin Anthony from New Jersey." What vitamin deficiency can cause this form of amnestic disorder?

a. Pantothenic acid
b. Folate
c. Thiamine
d. Riboflavin
e. Niacin

110. A 78-year-old man awakens from a nap in a state of great agitation. Although he appears to want to communicate, he only repeats the sentence "See you later" over and over. The right side of his face droops and he seems to have difficulties in lifting his right arm. A CAT scan shows a recent brain infarct. Where is the lesion most likely located?

a. Left parietal lobe
b. Right parietal lobe
c. Left frontal lobe
d. Right frontal lobe
e. Fronto-orbital region

Psychiatry

111. A 50-year-old man notes that several times per week he has a hallucination of the smell of burning rubber. He is diagnosed with partial complex seizures. Which of the following regions is most likely to show a discharging focus on EEG?
a. Parietal lobe
b. Temporal lobe
c. Frontal lobe
d. Thalamus
e. Occipital lobe

112. During a study on schizophrenia, a sample of children ages 12 to 15 years is recruited. Any child already showing signs of schizophrenia is excluded from the sample. Histories are taken looking for a variety of risk factors for developing schizophrenia. Every year thereafter, the children are evaluated to determine how many have developed schizophrenia. Which kind of study is this?
a. Clinical trial
b. Cohort study
c. Case-control study
d. Case-history study
e. Crossover study

113. Which of the following findings is associated with non-REM (NREM) sleep?
a. Penile tumescence
b. Apnea
c. Narcolepsy
d. Dreaming
e. Night terrors

114. A 17-year-old boy with a long history of aggressive behavior commits suicide by shooting himself with a gun. Analysis of his cerebrospinal fluid is likely to show an alteration in which of the following substances?
a. High levels of endorphins
b. Low levels of endorphins
c. High levels of serotonin
d. Low levels of serotonin
e. Low levels of substance P

115. A 34-year-old man comes to see a psychiatrist because he has been fired for constantly being late at his job. The man states he feels as if he is in danger of contamination from germs and as a result, he must take showers continuously, often for as many as 8 hours per day. Which of the following transmitters is thought to be involved in this disorder?
a. Dopamine
b. Norepinephrine
c. Acetylcholine
d. Histamine
e. Serotonin

Items 116–117

116. A 71-year-old man has been treated by a neurologist for Parkinson's disease for the past 2 years. One week after his last visit, he called his neurologist reporting that he suddenly began seeing little people walking all over his furniture. What is the most likely cause of this hallucination?
a. L-dopa was decreased at the last visit
b. The patient is delirious
c. L-dopa was increased at the last visit
d. The patient has developed a psychotic depression
e. The Parkinson's disease is worsening

117. What should the neurologist do with this patient?
a. Reduce the L-dopa
b. Increase the L-dopa
c. Add haloperidol
d. Add Sinemet
e. Call a psychiatrist for consultation

118. A 3-month-old girl is brought to the physician by her mother because she believes the child is deaf. On examination, the child also has bilateral cataracts, microcephaly, and microphthalmia. Which of the following organisms most likely infected this patient in utero?
a. *Escherichia coli*
b. Syphilis
c. Cytomegalovirus
d. Rubella
e. HIV

DIRECTIONS: Each group of questions below consists of lettered options followed by a set of numbered items. For each numbered item, select the **one** lettered option with which it is **most** closely associated. Each lettered option may be used once, more than once, or not at all.

Items 119–122

a. Glutamic acid
b. GABA
c. Norepinephrine
d. Somatostatin
e. Substance P
f. Glutamate
g. Acetylcholine
h. Serotonin

119. Which of the above substances is a catecholamine? **(CHOOSE 1 SUBSTANCE)**

120. Which of the above substances is an excitatory amino acid in the central nervous system? **(CHOOSE 1 SUBSTANCE)**

121. Which of the above substances is a neuropeptide? **(CHOOSE 1 SUBSTANCE)**

122. Which of the above substances is an inhibitory amino acid? **(CHOOSE 1 SUBSTANCE)**

123. A 43-year-old woman with a brain lesion develops a voracious appetite and bouts of rage. Where in the brain is the lesion located?
a. Ventromedial nucleus of the hypothalamus
b. Thalamic reticular activating system
c. Hypothalamus
d. Precentral guyrus
e. Mammillary bodies

124. Which of the following sites is thought to be significant for formation and storage of immediate and recent memories?

a. Hypothalamus
b. Nucleus basalis of Meynert
c. Mesolimbic circuit
d. Hippocampus
e. Amygdala

125. A 54-year-old man is a chronic alcoholic. He has been diagnosed with Korsakoff's syndrome (a severe inability to form new memories and a variable inability to recall remote memories). Where is the damage causing this memory loss located in the brain?

a. Angular gyrus
b. Mamillary bodies
c. Hypothalamus
d. Globus pallidus
e. Arcuate fasciculus

126. A 32-year-old woman had a car accident in which she incurred head trauma. After the accident, she is noted to be placid and hypersexual, quite unlike her preaccident behavior. She is also noted to have constantly shifting attention, and she places most objects given to her in her mouth. Where is the damage in her brain that is the cause of this behavior?

a. Temporal lobes
b. Frontal lobes
c. Parietal lobes
d. Occipital lobes
e. Prefrontal cortex

127. A 58-year-old man has a brain lesion that causes him to feel euphoric, laugh uncontrollably, and joke and make puns. Where is this brain lesion most likely located?

a. Fornix
b. Right prefrontal cortex
c. Hippocampus
d. Left orbitofrontal cortex
e. Amygdala

128. A 28-year-old man is noted to have disinhibition, lability, and euphoria. He is also noted to have a lack of remorse. Which area of the man's brain is likely to be dysfunctional?
a. Orbitofrontal region of frontal lobe
b. Dorsolateral region of frontal lobe
c. Medial region of frontal lobe
d. Limbic system
e. Parietal lobe

129. A 44-year-old man has had a traumatic injury to his brain. Since the accident he appears inattentive and undermotivated. He tends to linger on trivial thoughts and echoes the examiner's questions. Which area of the man's brain is likely to have been traumatized?
a. Orbitofrontal region of frontal lobe
b. Dorsolateral region of frontal lobe
c. Medial region of frontal lobe
d. Limbic system
e. Parietal lobe

Items 130–131

	Spontaneous Speech	Auditory Comprehension	Repetition	Naming
a.	Nonfluent	Good	Poor	Poor
b.	Nonfluent	Poor	Poor	Poor
c.	Nonfluent	Good	Good	Poor
d.	Fluent	Poor	Poor	Poor
e.	Fluent	Good	Poor	Poor

130. A 74-year-old woman is diagnosed with Broca's aphasia. Which of the above describes the characteristics of this disorder? **(CHOOSE 1 DESCRIPTION)**

131. A 65-year-old man has a lesion in Wernicke's area of his left hemisphere. Which of the above describes the aphasia syndrome he would demonstrate? **(CHOOSE 1 DESCRIPTION)**

132. A 48-year-old man with Huntington's disease has irregular, involuntary spasmodic movements of his limbs and facial muscles, as well as psychosis. In a postmortem autopsy, which structure in his brain will likely be markedly shrunken?

a. Cerebellum
b. Striatum
c. Putamen
d. Substantia nigra
e. Caudate nucleus

Human Behavior: Biologic and Related Sciences

Answers

94. The answer is a. *(Kaplan, 8/e, p 280.)* Cataplexy refers to a sudden loss of muscle tone (ranging in severity from weakness in the knee to a total loss of tone), triggered by strong emotions, that takes place during full wakefulness. Cataplexy is thought to be due to an abnormal intrusion of REM sleep phenomena in periods of wakefulness. It is usually treated with medications that reduce REM sleep, such as antidepressants. Cataplexy may be a symptom of narcolepsy, another dyssomnia characterized by the irresistible urge to fall asleep regardless of the situation.

95. The answer is b. *(Kaplan, 8/e, p 1153.)* When animals are exposed to prolonged and inescapable stress, they develop analgesia through the release of endogenous opiates such as endorphins. Equally, patients who have experienced severe trauma readily release opiates in response to any stimulus that is reminiscent of the original trauma. This release, in turn, causes psychic numbing, a subjective feeling of calm and analgesia. This response can be suppressed by opiate antagonists and explains why traumatized people use self-injury as a way to calm themselves.

96. The answer is e. *(Kaplan, 8/e, p 110.)* GABA receptors represent the most important inhibitory system in the central nervous system (CNS) and are found in almost every area the brain. Benzodiazepines, barbiturates, and many anticonvulsants act through activation of the GABA receptors. This explains the cross-tolerance that occurs between these substances.

97. The answer is b. *(Kaplan, 8/e, p 113.)* Levodopa is a chemical relative of dopamine. The fact that a dopamine-related compound can cause psychotic symptoms in some patients supports the dopamine hypothesis of schizophrenia, which is the leading neurochemical hypothesis for this disease.

98. The answer is a. *(Kaplan, 8/e, p 542.)* Seasonal circadian rhythm has been implicated in the etiology of seasonal affective disorder, which is characterized by a recurrent major depression that starts in November and resolves in March. Winter's short days cause a change in the pattern of secretion of nocturnal melatonin, which is inhibited by light. In animals, this causes a decrease in activity level, reproduction-related behaviors, and aggressive behavior. The same mechanism is postulated to be effective in seasonal depression, which, in fact, responds to light therapy.

99. The answer is e. *(Kaplan, 8/e, p 738.)* Dreaming is the main characteristic of rapid eye movement (REM) sleep. The EEG shows characteristic low-voltage waves that are random, fast, and sawtoothed. Active eye movements are attributed to the individual's "watching" his or her dreams. A lack of muscle tone during REM sleep prevents the individual from acting out his or her dreams. REM sleep is also characterized by increased heart rate and blood pressure and penile or clitoral nocturnal erections.

100. The answer is e. *(Kaplan, 8/e, p 94.)* The frontal lobes are associated with the regulation of emotions, the manifestation of behavioral traits usually connected to the personality of an individual, and executive functions (the ability to make appropriate judgments and decisions and to form concepts). They also contain the inhibitory systems for behaviors such as bladder and bowel release. Damage of the frontal lobes causes impairment of these functions but it is not, strictly speaking, a form of dementia, because memory, language, calculation ability, praxis, and IQ are often preserved. Personality changes, disinhibited behavior, and poor judgment are usually seen with lesions of the dorsolateral regions of the frontal lobes. Lesions of the mesial region, which is involved in the regulation of the initiation of movements and emotional responses, cause slowing of motor functions, speech, and emotional reactions. In the most severe cases, patients are mute and akinetic. Lesions of the orbitofrontal area are accompanied by abnormal social behaviors, an excessively good opinion of oneself, jocularity, sexual disinhibition, and lack of concern for others.

101. The answer is e. *(Kaplan, 8/e, p 1141.)* Prader-Willi syndrome is a genetic disorder caused by a defect of the long arm of chromosome 15. Characteristically, children are underweight in infancy. In early childhood, due to a hypothalamic dysfunction, they start eating voraciously and quickly become grossly overweight. Individuals with this syndrome have characteristic facial features and present with a variety of neurologic and neuropsychiatric symptoms including autonomic dysregulation; muscle weakness; hypotonia; mild to moderate mental retardation; temper tantrums; violent outbursts; perseveration; skin picking; and a tendency to be argumentative, oppositional, and rigid.

102. The answer is d. *(Kaplan, 8/e, p 1140.)* Fragile X syndrome is the most common form of inherited mental retardation, with a prevalence of 1 in 1200 in males and 1 in 2500 in females. Its manifestations are due to the inactivation of the fragile X mental retardation gene. Affected individuals have characteristic physical features including long face, large ears, and large hands. Adult males also have enlarged testicles due to elevated gonadotropin levels. Affected individuals and female carriers have higher rates of OCD, ADHD, dysthymia, anxiety, and antisocial personality disorder. Individuals with fragile X syndrome also display many behaviors reminiscent of autism. They are shy and socially awkward, they avoid eye contact, and, as autistic individuals, they engage in self-stimulatory, peculiar, and self-injurious behaviors. Down syndrome is the most common genetic mental retardation syndrome, occurring in 1 in 660 live births, but in the majority of cases (94%) it is due to a de novo trisomy of chromosome 21 and, as such, it is not inherited. Hurler's syndrome is one of the mucopolysaccharidoses. In its most severe form, this rare syndrome presents with multisystemic deterioration secondary to the accumulation of mucopolysaccharides. Hurler's syndrome starts during the first year of life and causes death before age 10. Rett's syndrome, a pervasive developmental disorder, is characterized by a devastating progressive deterioration of cognitive, social, and motor functions that starts between age 5 months and 18 months, after an initial period of normal development. Williams' syndrome is a rare form of genetic mental retardation caused by a deletion of part of chromosome 23.

103. The answer is b. *(Kaplan, 8/e, p 1061.)* Monoamine oxidases inactivate biogenic amines such as norepinephrine, serotonin, dopamine, and tyramine through oxidative deamination. The MAOIs block this inactivation, thereby increasing the availability of these neurotransmitters for synaptic release. Norepinephrine and serotonin play an important role in the pathophysiology of depression and other psychiatric disorders.

104. The answer is b. *(Kaplan, 8/e, p 122.)* A decreased latency of REM sleep is seen in major depression. Depression is the psychiatric disorder that has been most associated with disruptions in biological rhythms. Besides the decreased latency of REM sleep, one can find early morning awakening and other neuroendocrine perturbations.

105. The answer is e. *(Kaplan, 8/e, p 956.)* The boy in the question experienced an acute dystonic reaction, an adverse effect of neuroleptic medications secondary to blockage of dopamine receptors in the nigrostriatal system. Dystonic reactions are sustained spasmodic contractions of the muscles of the neck, trunk, tongue, face, and extraocular muscles. They can be quite painful and frightening. They usually occur within hours to 3 days after the beginning of the treatment and are more frequent in males and young people. They are also usually associated with high-potency neuroleptics. Occasionally, dystonic reactions are seen in young people who have ingested a neuroleptic medication, mistaking it for a drug of abuse. Administration of anticholinergic drugs provides rapid treatment of acute dystonia.

106. The answer is c. *(Kaplan, 8/e, p 819.)* The symptoms experienced by the woman in the question are diagnostic for hypothyroidism. Depressive symptoms are commonly associated with this disorder. Hypocalcemia and hypercortisolemia (associated with an elevated ACTH in Cushing's syndrome) are also associated with depression but present with different symptoms.

107. The answer is a. *(Kaplan, 8/e, p 422.)* Cocaine inhibits the normal reuptake of norepinephrine and dopamine, causing an increase of the concentration of these neurotransmitters in the synaptic cleft. This mechanism is responsible for the euphoria and sense of well-being that follow cocaine use, but it also causes excessive sympathetic activation and diffuse vasoconstriction. High blood pressure, mydriasis, cardiac arrhythmias, coronary artery spasms, and myocardial infarcts are all seen with cocaine intoxication. Other toxic effects of cocaine include headaches, ischemic cerebral and spinal infarcts, subarachnoid hemorrhages, and seizures.

Ritalin, heroin, PCP, and LSD intoxications present with different symptoms and signs.

108. The answer is a. *(Kaplan, 8/e, p 115.)* The cell bodies of serotonin-releasing neurons are located in the midbrain in a group of nuclei called the raphe nuclei. Through their projections to virtually all areas of the central nervous system, the raphe nuclei contribute to the regulation of mood, sleep, pain transmission, and aggression.

109. The answer is c. *(Kaplan, 8/e, p 363.)* Severe anterograde memory deficits with an inability to form new memories are the main feature of Korsakoff's syndrome or alcohol-induced persisting amnestic disorder. Retrograde amnesia is also present, with the most severe loss of memory occurring for events that were closer to the beginning of the disorder. Remote memories are relatively preserved. The disorder is due to dietary thiamine deficiency and subsequent damage of the thiamine-dependent structures of the brain (mammillary bodies and the regions surrounding the third and fourth ventricles). Korsakoff's syndrome can sometimes (though rarely) be due to other causes of thiamine deficiency, such as diseases that cause severe malabsorption.

110. The answer is c. *(Kaplan, 8/e, p 92.)* Lesions of the Broca area, located in most right-handed people in the left frontal lobe, cause nonfluent aphasia, a disorder characterized by a severe reduction of speech with normal comprehension. Speech is limited to single words or repetition of one or two common sentences. The most common cause is a stroke in the middle cerebral artery territory. Right hemiparesis with a particular involvement of the lower face and the arm and dysarthria are usually associated features, due to the proximity of the parietal primary motor area. Nonfluent aphasia can be confused with delirium or psychosis due to the unusual speech production and the patient's acute distress and agitation.

111. The answer is b. *(Goldman, 5/e, p 140.)* Partial complex seizures usually (90% of the time) originate from the temporal lobe. Auras that consist of unpleasant odors often originate from the uncus, an area at the tip of the temporal lobe that is involved in processing olfactory sensations. In the past, such seizures were called uncinate fits.

Human Behavior: Biologic and Related Sciences *Answers* **75**

112. The answer is b. *(Kaplan, 8/e, p 172.)* A cohort study is a group chosen from a well-defined population that is studied over a long time. Cohort studies are also known as longitudinal studies. Cohort studies provide direct estimates of risk associated with a suspected causal factor.

113. The answer is e. *(Kaplan, 8/e, p 754.)* Night terrors are characterized by a partial awakening accompanied by screaming, thrashing, and autonomic arousal. They are non-REM sleep events. Increase in blood pressure and heart rate, penile erection, and dreaming are associated with REM sleep.

114. The answer is d. *(Kaplan, 8/e, p 159.)* The correlation between low levels of serotonin in the cerebrospinal fluid (CSF) and aggressive behavior has been proved by many studies conducted with animals and human subjects. There is a clear inverse relationship between the levels of CSF serotonin in both violent suicidal behavior in depressed patients and aggressive behavior in patients with personality disorders. Endorphins and substance P are involved in the transmission and modulation of pain.

115. The answer is e. *(Kaplan, 8/e, p 610.)* It has been proven that a dysfunction of serotoninergic pathways is implicated in the genesis of obsessive-compulsive disorder. This finding is supported by the antiobsessional effects of medications that increase the concentration of serotonin in the synaptic cleft, such as SSRIs and clomipramine (a tricyclic). Of the other neurotransmitters, dopamine is linked to psychosis, acetylcholine plays a role in cognitive functions and memory, and norepinephrine is involved in anxiety disorders.

116–117. The answers are 116-c, 117-a. *(Kaplan, 8/e, p 1045.)* Hallucinations are the most common side effect of anti-Parkinson's medications. Hallucinations occur in 30% of the treated patients and can be induced by any type of medication used to treat Parkinson's disease, including dopaminergic agents such as L-dopa and amantidine, MAO inhibitors, and anticholinergic medications. The hallucinations usually consist of clear images of people and animals and may be preceded by sleep disturbances. Increasing age, polypharmacy, long treatment, and use of anticholinergic medications increase the risk for developing hallucinations. Reducing the dosage or eliminating anticholinergic agents is usually the only necessary treatment.

118. The answer is d. *(Kaplan, 8/e, p 1146.)* Rubella is the major cause of congenital malformations and mental retardation owing to maternal infection. The children of affected mothers may show several abnormalities, including congenital heart disease, mental retardation, cataracts, deafness, microcephaly, and microphthalmia. Timing is crucial, as the extent and the frequency of the complications are inversely related to the duration of the pregnancy at the time of the maternal infection. Maternal rubella can be prevented by immunization.

119–122. The answers are 119-c, 120-f, 121-e, 122-b. *(Kaplan, 8/e, pp 113, 109, 118, 1110.)* CNS neurotransmitters include amino acids, biogenic amines, and neuropeptides. There are many other neurotransmitter substances, and many are still poorly understood. This is one of the most exciting areas of current psychiatric research. As more and more knowledge accrues, it becomes possible to develop more specific psychopharmacologic interventions. Glutamic and aspartic acids have excitatory properties. GABA is the principal inhibitory neurotransmitter. The biogenic amines include the catecholamines such as dopamine, norepinephrine, epinephrine, histamine, and the indolamine serotonin. Neuropeptides include β-endorphin, somatostatin, and vasopressin, and substance P.

123. The answer is a. *(Kaplan, 8/e, p 88.)* The brain center that drives the autonomic motor system is the hypothalamus, which houses a set of paired nuclei that appear to control appetite, rage, temperature, blood pressure, perspiration, and sexual drive. Lesions to the ventromedial nucleus of the hypothalamus—the satiety center—produce a voracious appetite and rage.

124. The answer is d. *(Kaplan, 8/e, p 91.)* Data from a series of animal experiments suggest that the hippocampus is the site for formation and storage of immediate and recent memories. It is even thought (though no data yet support this) that the hippocampal map is inappropriately reactivated during a déjà vu experience.

125. The answer is b. *(Kaplan, 8/e, p 91.)* Within the diencephalon, the dorsal medial nucleus of the thalamus and the mamillary bodies appear necessary for memory formation. These two structures are damaged in thiamine-deficient states usually seen in chronic alcoholics, and their inactivation is associated with Korsakoff's syndrome.

Human Behavior: Biologic and Related Sciences *Answers* 77

126. The answer is a. (*Kaplan, 8/e, p 93.*) Bilateral injury to the temporal lobes can occur after head trauma, cardiac arrest, herpes simplex encephalitis, or in Pick's disease. This lesion resembles the one described in the Klüver-Bucy syndrome, an experimental model of temporal lobe ablation in monkeys. Behavior in this syndrome is characterized by hypersexuality, placidity, a tendency to explore the environment with the mouth, inability to recognize the emotional significance of visual stimuli, and constantly shifting attention, called hypermetamorphosis.

127. The answer is b. (*Kaplan, 8/e, p 93.*) A lesion to the left prefrontal area abolishes the normal mood-elevating influences of this area and produces depression and uncontrollable crying. In contrast, a comparable lesion to the right prefrontal area may produce laughter, euphoria, and a tendency to joke and make puns.

128. The answer is a. (*Kaplan, 8/e, p 95.*) Dysfunction of the orbitofrontal area causes disinhibition, irritability, lability, euphoria, and lack of remorse. Insight and judgement are impaired; patients are distractible. These features are reminiscent of the diagnoses of antisocial personality disorder, intermittent explosive disorder, and episodic dyscontrol syndrome.

129. The answer is b. (*Kaplan, 8/e, p 95.*) Lesions in the dorsolateral area lead to deficiencies of planning, monitoring, flexibility, and motivation. Patients may be unable to use foresight and feedback or to maintain goal-directedness, focus, or sustained effort. They appear inattentive and under-motivated, cannot plan novel cognitive activity, and exhibit a tendency to linger on trivial thoughts. They may echo the examiner's questions and react primarily to details of environmental stimuli—missing the forest for the trees.

130–131. The answers are 130-a, 131-d. (*Kaplan, 8/e, p 89.*) Broca's aphasia, a loss of fluent speech caused by a lesion in the left inferior frontal lobe, was described by Broca in 1865. While all fluent speech is lost (and thus the ability to repeat and name is poor), auditory comprehension remains intact. Wernicke localized language comprehension to the left superior temporal lobe in 1874. In this aphasia, language is not comprehended, so repetition and naming are poor. The patient's speech remains fluent however.

132. The answer is e. *(Kaplan, 8/e, p 87.)* The caudate nucleus plays an important role in the modulation of motor acts. When functioning properly, the caudate acts as a gatekeeper to allow the motor system to perform only those acts that are goal-directed. When it fails, extraneous acts are performed. The caudate shrinks dramatically in Huntington's disease. The disorder is characterized by rigidity, on which is gradually superimposed choreiform or "dancing" movements.

Disorders of Childhood and Adolescence

Questions

DIRECTIONS: Each item below contains a question or incomplete statement followed by suggested responses. Select the **one best** response to each question.

133. A 5-year-old boy is brought to the psychiatrist because he has difficulty paying attention in school. He fidgets and squirms and will not stay seated in class. At home he is noted to talk excessively and has difficulty waiting for his turn. His language and motor skills are appropriate for his age. Which of the following is most likely this child's diagnosis?
a. Oppositional defiant disorder (ODD)
b. Attention-deficit/hyperactivity disorder (ADHD)
c. Pervasive developmental disorder
d. Separation anxiety disorder
e. Mild mental retardation

134. A 7-year-old boy with an IQ of 65 due to fragile X syndrome is brought to a psychiatrist because he has been fidgeting, increasingly restless, and unable to focus. He cannot sit still for more than a minute or two. The teachers in his special education school report similar difficulties in the classroom. What percentage of mentally retarded children also exhibit these symptoms?
a. 0 to 3%
b. 10 to 20%
c. 30 to 40%
d. 50 to 60%
e. 75 to 85%

135. The parents of an 8-year-old boy with a normal IQ are concerned because he is a very slow reader and does not appear to understand what he reads. When the boy reads aloud, he misses words and changes the sequence of the letters. Which of the following statements is true about this disorder?

a. It is diagnosed on the basis of a defect in visual or hearing acuity
b. It is often associated with spelling and verbal language difficulties
c. It occurs in less than 1% of the population
d. Children usually grow out of the disorder when adulthood is reached
e. It is often associated with brainstem neurologic defects

136. For the past 3 months, a 15-year-old girl has had to turn her light on and off 23 times at exactly 10:30 P.M. before she can go to bed. She can spend from 1 to 2 h on this ritual because she has to start again if she is interrupted or loses count. She is upset if the position of the order of the objects she has on her desk is changed even slightly and cannot stop worrying about her family's safety. In conjunction with pharmacologic treatment, which therapy has been proven effective for this disorder?

a. Play therapy
b. Psychodynamic psychotherapy
c. Group therapy
d. Cognitive-behavioral therapy
e. Family therapy

137. A 9-year-old boy from a single-parent household is mandated to attend a fire prevention group after setting fire to a toolshed in his backyard. The boy began by setting a small pile of leaves on fire, then he poured gasoline on it. The fire went out of control and engulfed the toolshed. The boy's mother reports to the police that there have been at least four previous fire-setting incidents during the previous 6 months. Which of the following statements is true about this disorder?

a. Girls and boys are equally at risk for pathological fire setting
b. Fires started by children rarely cause any serious damage
c. Children younger than 6 are not likely to experiment with fire
d. The prognosis for treated children is excellent
e. A commonly associated feature is a lower-than-average IQ

138. A 5-year-old is being evaluated for ADHD. He has a past history of failure to thrive and he is still at the fifteenth percentile for weight and height. The evaluator notices that he has unusually small eyes with short palpebral fissures as well as a thin upper lip with a smooth philtrum. Which substance did his mother abuse during pregnancy?
a. Heroin
b. Nicotine
c. Cannabis
d. Alcohol
e. Cocaine

139. A 7-year-old boy avoids having sleepovers because he wets his bed almost every night and is afraid his friends would tease him. Which of the following statements is true about this disorder?
a. It is diagnosed before the age of 5
b. It is more common in girls than boys
c. It has a strong genetic component
d. Spontaneous remissions almost never occur
e. For many children, the disorder is ego-syntonic

140. A 13-year-old girl grunts and clears her throat several times in an hour, and her conversation is often interrupted by random shouting. She also performs idiosyncratic, complex motor activities such as turning her head to the right while she shuts her eyes and opens her mouth. She can prevent these movements for brief periods of time, with effort. Which of the following is the most appropriate treatment for this disorder?
a. Individual psychodynamic psychotherapy
b. Lorazepam
c. Methylphenidate
d. Haloperidol
e. Imipramine

141. A 6-year-old boy has been diagnosed with ADHD and started on Ritalin. Which of the following serious side effects should the child psychiatrist warn the boy's parents about?
a. Tics
b. Cardiac conduction abnormalities
c. Choreiform movements
d. Leukopenia
e. Hepatitis

142. Every morning on school days, an 8-year-old girl becomes tearful and distressed and claims she feels sick. Once in school, she often goes to the nurse, complaining of headaches and stomach pains. At least once a week, she misses school or is picked up early by her mother due to her complaints. Her pediatrician has ruled out organic causes for the physical symptoms. The child is usually symptom free on weekends, unless her parents go out and leave her with a baby sitter. Which of the following is the most likely diagnosis?
a. Separation anxiety disorder
b. Major depression
c. Somatization disorder
d. Generalized anxiety disorder
e. Attachment disorder

143. A 1-year-old girl has been hospitalized on numerous occasions for periods of apnea. Each time her mother had called an ambulance after her daughter had stopped breathing suddenly. All workups in the hospital have been negative, and the patient has never had an episode in front of anyone but her mother. Although the patient's mother seems very involved with the child and the staff on the unit, she does not seem hesitant about consenting to lab tests on her daughter, even if the tests are invasive. Which of the following statements is true about this disorder?
a. It is usually self-limited
b. The father is usually the perpetrator
c. It is a form of child abuse
d. Usually only one child is victimized in a family
e. The motivation is watching the child suffer

144. A social worker makes a routine visit on a 3-year-old boy who has just been returned to his biological mother after spending 3 months in foster care for severe neglect. The child initially appears very shy and clings fearfully to his mother. Later on, he starts playing in a very destructive and disorganized way. When the mother tries to stop him from throwing blocks at her, he starts kicking and biting. The mother becomes enraged and starts shouting. Which of the following is most likely to be this child's diagnosis?
a. Oppositional defiant disorder
b. ADHD
c. Reactive attachment disorder
d. PTSD
e. Major depression

145. A first-grade teacher is concerned about a 6-year-old girl in her class who has not spoken a single word since school started. The little girl participates appropriately in the class activities and uses gestures and drawings and nods and shakes her head to communicate. The parents report that the little girl talks only in the home and only in the presence of her closest relatives. Which of the following is the most appropriate diagnosis?

a. Autism
b. Expressive language disorder
c. Oppositional defiant disorder
d. School phobia
e. Selective mutism

146. A 4-year-old boy is brought to the physician by his parents for episodes of waking in the middle of the night screaming. The parents state that when they get to the boy's room during one of these episodes, they find him in his bed, thrashing wildly, his eyes wide open. He pushes them away when they try to comfort him. After 2 min, the boy suddenly falls asleep, and the next day he has no memory of the episode. Which of the following medications is used to treat this disorder?

a. Haloperidol
b. Diazepam
c. Methylphenidate
d. Amitryptiline
e. Valproic acid

147. A 14-year-old boy is brought to the physician because he told his mother he wished he were dead. He has been irritable for the past several weeks, and has been isolating himself in his room, avoiding his friends. He has been complaining of general aches and pains as well. Which of the following statements is true about this disorder?

a. It is rare in children
b. Its presentation in children is similar to that in adults
c. Medications are not the treatment of choice
d. Psychotic symptoms are common
e. Questions about suicide will increase the likelihood of self-destructive behavior

148. The flow of a 5-year-old boy's speech is interrupted by hesitations, repetition of syllables, and excessive sound prolongations. These symptoms worsen when the boy is asked to speak in front of the class. Which of the following statements about this disorder is correct?

a. It typically worsens with anxiety
b. It usually starts between the ages of 10 and 13
c. Treatment predominantly involves the use of medication
d. It is commonly associated with major mental illness
e. Family members are rarely affected

149. A 5-year-old boy does not show any interest in other children and ignores adults other than his parents. He spends hours lining up his toy cars or spinning their wheels but does not use them for "make-believe" play. He rarely uses speech to communicate. Which of the following diagnoses is most likely in this boy?

a. Major depression
b. Mental retardation
c. ADHD
d. Autism
e. Conduct disorder

150. A 15-year-old boy is arrested for shooting the owner of the convenience store he tried to rob. He has been in Department of Youth Services custody several times for a variety of crimes against property, possession of illegal substances, and assault and battery. He is cheerful and unconcerned during the arrest, more worried about not losing his leather jacket than about the fate of the man he has injured. Which of the following is the most appropriate diagnosis in this case?

a. Oppositional defiant disorder
b. Antisocial personality disorder
c. Narcissistic personality disorder
d. Conduct disorder
e. Substance abuse

Disorders of Childhood and Adolescence

Answers

133. The answer is b. *(Kaplan, 8/e, p 576.)* Excessive motor activity, usually with intrusive and annoying qualities, poor sustained attention, difficulties inhibiting impulsive behaviors in social situations and on cognitive tasks, and difficulties with peers are the main characteristics of ADHD, combined type. Symptoms must be present in two or more settings (in this case, home and school) and must cause significant impairment.

134. The answer is b. *(Stoudemire, 3/e, p 585.)* Rates of ADHD in mentally retarded children range from 10 to 20%. Stimulants are as effective in mentally retarded children with ADHD as in children with normal intelligence, but the incidence of tics and emotional withdrawal may be higher. Emotional and psychiatric disorders are more common in mentally retarded than in nonretarded individuals. In Rutter's Isle of Wight study, 30 to 40% of the children with an IQ lower than 75 were found to have psychiatric disorders. In the nonretarded population, by comparison, rates were between 7.7 and 9.5%.

135. The answer is b. *(Stoudemire, 3/e, p 590.)* Dyslexia occurs in 3 to 10% of the population. When a reading disorder is caused by a defect in visual or hearing acuity, it is excluded by diagnostic criteria from the diagnosis of developmental reading disorder. Almost all patients with this problem have spelling difficulties, and nearly all have verbal language defects. Children do not grow out of the disorder by adulthood. It is believed that the most common etiology relates to cortical brain pathology.

136. The answer is d. *(Stoudemire, 3/e, p 556.)* Behavioral therapy techniques such as exposure and response prevention and desensitization are very effective in adults and adolescents with a diagnosis of OCD. OCD has a lifetime prevalence of between 0.2 and 1.2% in children. Children as young as 2 have been diagnosed with the disorder. Contrary to the case in adult-onset OCD, obsessions and compulsion are often ego-syntonic in childhood OCD.

137. The answer is e. *(Kaplan, 8/e, p 764.)* Most children between ages 3 and 5 show an interest in fire. Experimentation with matches or other incendiary materials emerges between 5 and 9 years of age. Boys are more likely to start fires than girls. Inattention, impulsivity, poor school performance, learning disability, mental retardation, and decreased ability to modulate anger are more frequent in fire setters than in the general population. Single-parent homes; conflicted, cold, and negative family interactions; and a greater use of harsh physical discipline are frequent in the history of fire setters. Fires started by children cause many deaths and injuries and serious economic damage each year. In 1991, children started 103,260 fires that caused 457 deaths, 1,856 injuries, and $310 million in property damage. Fire setting is the leading cause of death for preschoolers and the second leading cause of death (after automobile accidents) for children between 6 and 14. While younger children set fires alone, adolescents do so with friends, usually in the context of a peer group that encourages or condones this and other deviant behaviors. Little has been written about the treatment of pyromania, and fire setters are typically difficult to treat because of their lack of motivation.

138. The answer is d. *(Stoudemire, 3/e, p 396.)* Fetal alcohol syndrome occurs in 1 to 2 live births per 1000, and among 2 to 10% of alcoholic mothers. Fetal alcohol syndrome is characterized by intrauterine growth retardation and persistent postnatal poor growth, microcephaly, developmental delays, attentional deficits, learning disabilities, and hyperactivity. Characteristic facial features are microphthalmia with short palpebral fissures, midface hypoplasia, thin upper lip, and a smooth and/or long philtrum. Children whose mothers used opiates during pregnancy are born passively addicted to the drugs and exhibit withdrawal symptoms in the first days and weeks of life. During the first year of life, these infants show poor motor coordination, hyperactivity, and inattention. These problems persist during school-age years, although few differences in cognitive performance are reported. Infants exposed to cannabis prenatally present with decreased visual responsiveness, tremor, increased startle reflex, and disrupted sleep patterns. Long-term longitudinal outcome studies are few and contradictory. Prenatal exposure to cocaine causes impaired startle response; impaired habituation, recognition, and reactivity to novel stimuli; and increased irritability in infants. Older children present with language delays, poor motor coordination, hyperactivity, and attentional deficits.

139. The answer is c. *(Kaplan, 8/e, p 1226.)* About 75% of enuretic children have a first-degree relative who is or was enuretic. A child's risk for enuresis has been found to be more than 7 times greater if the father was enuretic. Nocturnal enuresis is not diagnosed before age 5, an age at which continence is usually expected. The incidence in boys is somewhat higher than in girls. This disorder is often associated with daytime (diurnal) wetting. Nocturnal enuresis usually is diagnosed in childhood, although adolescent onset does occur. When the disorder starts in adolescence, it tends to be associated with more psychopathology and to have a poorer prognosis. Nocturnal enuresis usually occurs 30 min to 3 h after the onset of sleep. About half of enuretic children have other associated emotional disturbances, though it is sometimes difficult to separate cause and effect. Enuresis is usually self-limited. Most enuretic children find their symptoms ego-dystonic and have enhanced self-esteem and improved social confidence when they become continent.

140. The answer is d. *(Stoudemire, 3/e, p 579.)* Vocal tics such as grunting, barking, throat clearing, coprolalia (the repetitive speaking of vulgarities), and shouting and simple and complex motor tics are characteristic findings of Tourette's syndrome. Pharmacological treatment of this disorder includes neuroleptics and α_2 agonists (clonidine, guanfacine).

141. The answer is a. *(Ebert, p 526.)* Common side effects of methylphenidate include loss of appetite and weight, irritability, oversensitivity and crying spells, headaches, and abdominal pain. Insomnia may occur, particularly when this agent is dispensed late in the day. Tics, while a less frequent complication of stimulant treatment, can cause significant impairment. Choreiform movements and night terrors are side effects of another stimulant, pemoline. Leukopenia, hepatitis, and cardiac arrhythmias are not associated with stimulant treatment.

142. The answer is a. *(Ebert, p 579.)* Separation anxiety disorder is characterized by manifestations of distress when the child has to be separated from loved ones. The distress often leads to school refusal, refusal to sleep alone, multiple somatic symptoms, and complaints when the child is separated from loved ones, and at times may be associated with full-blown panic attacks. The child is typically afraid that harm will come either to loved ones or to him- or herself during the time of separation. This is normal behavior in children 1 to 3 years old, after which it is thought to be pathological.

143. The answer is c. (*Ebert, p 380.*) In Munchausen syndrome by proxy, a caregiver, usually the mother, fabricates or produces symptoms of illness in a child. The caregiver's motive is to vicariously receive care and attention from health providers through the sick child. The severity of the disorder varies from cases in which symptoms are completely fabricated to cases in which the mother causes serious physical damage or even death to the child. Mothers with Munchhausen by proxy are extremely attentive to their children and often are considered model parents. These mothers are not cognitively impaired or psychotic; on the contrary, they are often quite accomplished and knowledgeable and frequently work or have worked in the medical field. Not infrequently, more than one child is victimized in a family, particularly in cases of suffocation disguised as sudden infant death syndrome (SIDS) or apnea. A very pathological relationship develops between the mother and the victimized child, to the point that older children often collude with the mother in producing the symptoms.

144. The answer is c. (*Kaplan, 8/e, p 1237.*) Reactive attachment disorder is the product of a severely dysfunctional early relationship between the principal caregiver and the child. When caregivers consistently disregard the child's physical or emotional needs, the child fails to develop a secure and stable attachment with them. This failure causes a severe disturbance of the child's ability to relate to others, manifested in a variety of behavioral and interpersonal problems. Some children are fearful, inhibited, withdrawn, and apathetic; others are aggressive, disruptive, and disorganized with low frustration tolerance and poor affect modulation. This condition is often confused with ODD or ADHD.

145. The answer is e. (*Kaplan, 8/e, p 1235.*) In selective mutism, a child voluntarily abstains from talking in particular situations (usually at school) while remaining appropriately verbal at home. Some children only speak with their parents and siblings and are mute with relatives and friends.

Children with selective mutism do not have a language impediment, nor do they display the lack of social interactions, lack of imagination, and stereotyped behavior characteristic of autism. On the contrary, they can be quite interactive and communicative in a nonverbal way, using drawing, writing, and pantomime. Children with school phobia refuse to go to school but do not have problems communicating through language. Oppositional defiant disorder is characterized by persistent refusal to follow rules and defiance toward authorities, not by failure to speak.

146. The answer is b. *(Kaplan, 8/e, p 754.)* The child in the question is experiencing episodes of sleep terror disorder, a dyssomnia characterized by sudden partial arousal accompanied by piercing screams, motor agitation, disorientation, and autonomic arousal. The episodes take place during the transition from deep sleep to REM sleep. Children do not report nightmares (which would be associated with REM sleep) and do not have any memory of the episodes the next day. Sleep terrors occur in 3% of children and 1% of adults. Although specific treatment for this disorder is seldom required, in rare cases it is necessary. Diazepam (Valium) in small doses at bedtime improves the condition and sometimes completely eliminates the attacks.

147. The answer is d. *(Stoudemire, 3/e, p 565.)* Depressive disorders are not rare in children, and often children with depression have relatives who also suffer from depression or another mood disorder. The incidence of depression is estimated to be 0.9% in preschoolers, 1.9% in school-age children, and 4.7% in adolescents. The incidence is considerably higher among children with neurological or medical illnesses. The diagnosis can be difficult because younger children's symptoms differ from the symptoms of depression usually displayed by adults. Often, aggression and irritability replace sad affect, and poor school functioning or refusal to go to school may be the prominent manifestations. Psychotic symptoms are present in one-third of cases of childhood major depression. Asking a child about suicidal ideation does not increase the risk of the child acting on this wish.

148. The answer is a. *(Kaplan, 8/e, p 1175.)* The boy in the vignette presents with classic symptoms of stuttering. This disorder affects 2 to 4% of children, with a male predominance of 3:1 to 4:1. It tends to be most common in young children and usually resolves in older children and adults.

Genetic factors are very significant in stuttering, and the incidence of the disorder in relatives of affected persons is higher than that in the general population. Stuttering is not associated with any major mental illness. Anxiety does occur around situations where the individual is required to speak in public or social situations, and this can worsen the stuttering, which sometimes leads to restriction of lifestyle and avoidance of such situations. Speech therapy is considered the most successful treatment for stuttering.

149. The answer is d. *(Ebert, p 547.)* Autistic disorder is characterized by lack of interest in social interactions, severely impaired verbal and nonverbal communication, stereotyped behaviors, and a very restricted range of interests. Children with autism do not involve themselves in imaginative and imitative play and can spend hours lining and spinning things or dismantling toys and putting them together. Mentally retarded children are developmentally delayed, but their social interaction and interest in people are appropriate for their mental age. Children with conduct disorder display a persistent disregard for rules and other people's rights.

150. The answer is d. *(Ebert, p 570.)* Children with conduct disorder display a persistent disregard for rules and other people's rights that lasts at least 1 year. Aggression toward people and animals, destruction of property, deceit and illegal activities, and frequent truancy from school are the main characteristics of the disorder. Approximately one-third of children diagnosed with conduct disorder proceed to become delinquent adolescents, and many are diagnosed with antisocial personality disorder in adulthood. Patients with antisocial personality disorder display a pervasive pattern of disregard for and violation of the rights of others since the age of 15 years, with evidence of a conduct disorder before age 15. Substance abuse is just one facet of conduct disorder. Children with oppositional defiant disorder are problematic and rebellious but do not routinely engage in aggressive, destructive, or illegal activities. Also, they do not present with the lack of empathy for others and the disregard for other people's rights that are typical of conduct disorder.

Cognitive Disorders and Consultation-Liaison Psychiatry

Questions

DIRECTIONS: Each item below contains a question or incomplete statement followed by suggested responses. Select the **one best** response to each question.

151. For the past 10 years, the memory of a 74-year-old woman has progressively declined. Lately, she has caused several small kitchen fires by forgetting to turn off the stove, she cannot remember how to cook her favorite recipes, and she becomes disoriented and confused at night. She identifies an increasing number of objects as "that thing" because she cannot recall the correct name. Her muscle strength and balance are intact. Which of the following is the most likely diagnosis?

a. Huntington's disease
b. Multi-infarct dementia
c. Creutzfeldt-Jakob disease
d. Alzheimer's disease
e. Wilson's disease

152. A 70-year-old man with a dementing disorder dies in a car accident. During the previous 5 years, his personality had dramatically changed and he had caused much embarrassment to his family due to his intrusive and inappropriate behavior. Pathological examination of his brain shows frontotemporal atrophy, gliosis of the frontal lobes' white matter, characteristic intracellular inclusions, and swollen neurons. Amyloid plaques and neurofibrillary tangles are absent. Which of the following is the correct diagnosis?

a. Alzheimer's disease
b. Pick's disease
c. Creutzfeldt-Jakob disease
d. B_{12} deficiency dementia
e. HIV dementia

153. A 24-year-old previously healthy man is brought to the emergency room after he began yelling that people on the bus were out to hurt him. In the emergency room, he is agitated, hypervigilant, and anxious. He is unable to give much history other than to say that he is a graduate student and nothing like this has ever happened before. What is the most likely cause of this behavior?

a. Delirium
b. Pick's disease
c. Dissociative disorder
d. Vitamin B_{12} deficiency
e. Cocaine intoxication

154. An emaciated and lethargic 16-year-old girl arrives at the emergency room. Her blood pressure is 75/50, her heart rate is 52/min, her potassium is 2.8 mEq/L, and her bicarbonate is 40 mEq/L. The girl's parents report that she has lost 35 lb in 3 months but is still convinced that she is overweight. She eats only very small amounts of low-calorie food, and she runs 2 to 3 h every day. What other activities is this patient like to have engaged in?

a. Sexual promiscuity
b. Ethanol abuse
c. Purging
d. Wearing tight clothes
e. Shoplifting

155. A 69-year-old woman slips on the ice and hits her head on the pavement. During the following 3 weeks, she develops a persistent headache, is increasingly distractible and forgetful, and becomes fearful and disoriented at night. Which of the following is the most likely cause of these changes?

a. Subdural hematoma
b. Frontal lobe meningioma
c. Korsakoff's disease
d. Epidural hematoma
e. Multi-infarct dementia

Cognitive Disorders and Consultation-Liaison Psychiatry 93

156. A 43-year-old man is admitted to the neurology service after he went blind suddenly the morning of admission. The patient does not seem overly concerned with his sudden lack of vision. The only time he gets upset during the interview is when discussing his mother's recent death in Mexico—he was to bring his mother to the USA, but did not because he had been using drugs and did not save the needed money. Physical exam is completely negative. Which of the following diagnoses is most likely?
a. Conversion disorder
b. Hypochondriasis
c. Factitious disorder
d. Malingering
e. Delusional disorder

157. A 52-year-old man is diagnosed with Parkinson's disease. Which of the following statements is true?
a. Transmagnetic stimulation could improve his symptoms for 12 months
b. Psychotic symptoms are common in newly diagnosed patients
c. Patients with Parkinson's have a high comorbidity with affective disorders
d. High-potency neuroleptics are the treatment of choice
e. Antiparkinsonian drugs commonly cause mania

158. A 24-year-old man smells burnt rubber, then turns his head and upper body to the right, makes chewing movements, and fumbles with his clothes. During the episode, which lasts 1 min, he appears dazed. Which of the following is the most appropriate diagnosis?
a. Frontal lobe tumor
b. Derealization disorder
c. Conversion disorder
d. Absence seizure
e. Partial complex seizure

159. A 55-year-old man comes to the physician with the chief complaint of daytime drowsiness. He states that although he goes to bed at 10 P.M. and doesn't get up until 6 A.M., he is chronically tired and must take naps during the day. He wakes up in the morning with a headache and a dry mouth. His wife states he snores loudly. Which of the following is the most appropriate diagnosis?
   a. Obstructive sleep apnea
   b. Narcolepsy
   c. Central apnea
   d. Recurrent hypersomnia
   e. Major depression

160. A 35-year-old woman is diagnosed with widely metastatic breast cancer. After she is told the diagnosis, she calmly asks a few questions, then schedules a return appointment. She tells her husband at home that night that she has a "mild problem" that needn't worry him. Which of the following Kübler-Ross stages is this patient in?
   a. Anger
   b. Denial
   c. Sublimation
   d. Bargaining
   e. Acceptance

161. A 24-year-old woman is hospitalized after a suicide gesture in which she superficially slashed both her wrists. At the team meeting 3 days later, the male resident argues that the patient has been doing quite well, seems to be responding to therapy, and should be allowed to go on a pass. The nursing staff angrily argues that the resident is showing favoritism to the patient, and, because of her poor compliance with the unit rules, she should not be allowed out. The resident insists the nurses are being punitive. The defense mechanism being used by the patient in this scenario is a feature of which of the following personality disorders?
   a. Narcissistic
   b. Histrionic
   c. Borderline
   d. Antisocial
   e. Dependent

162. A 45-year-old woman who has been on chronic steroid treatment for her asthma has thin arms and legs but has a large amount of fat deposited on her abdomen, chest, and shoulders. Her skin is thin and atrophic, and she bruises easily. She has purple striae on her abdomen. Physical examination shows an elevated blood pressure, and lab tests show a decreased glucose tolerance. Which of the following psychiatric diagnoses is most likely?

a. Major depression
b. Bipolar-mania
c. Substance-induced mood disorder
d. Delirium
e. Schizoaffective disorder

163. During the past year, a 25-year-old woman has had two episodes of diplopia and one episode of unilateral blindness that resolved spontaneously in a few weeks. She presents to her neurologist complaining of right arm weakness and urinary incontinence. Her MRI shows areas of hyperdensity localized in the white matter. The neurologist asks her many detailed questions about her mood, memory, and concentration. What is the most likely reason for such inquiry?

a. The patient may have a conversion disorder
b. The patient's neurological disorder is frequently accompanied by psychiatric symptoms
c. The physician is worried about the patient's potential for suicidality
d. The patient may be malingering
e. The patient may have a mood disorder secondary to a general medical condition

164. A 34-year-old man recurrently perceives the smell of rotten eggs. This kind of hallucination is most commonly seen in patients with which of the following diagnoses?

a. Parietal tumors
b. Narcolepsy
c. Grand mal epilepsy
d. Partial complex seizures
e. Wilson's disease

165. A 40-year-old woman's cognitive functions have progressively deteriorated for several years, to the point where she needs nursing home–level care. She is depressed, easily irritated, and prone to aggressive outbursts, a dramatic change from her premorbid personality. She also presents with irregular, purposeless, and asymmetrical movements of her face, limbs, and trunk, which worsen when she is upset and disappear in sleep. Her MRI shows atrophy of the caudal nucleus and the putamen. Which of the following diagnoses is most likely in this patient?

a. Creutzfeldt-Jakob disease
b. Wilson's disease
c. Huntington's disease
d. Alzheimer's disease
e. Multi-infarct dementia

166. A 37-year-old mildly retarded man with trisomy 21 syndrome has been increasingly forgetful. He makes frequent mistakes when counting change at the grocery store where he has worked for several years. In the past, he used to perform this task without difficulties. He often cannot recall the names of common objects, and he has started annoying customers with his intrusive questions. Which of the following diagnoses is most likely in this patient?

a. Pseudodementia
b. Hypothalamic tumor
c. Alzheimer's disease
d. Wilson's disease
e. Thiamine deficiency

167. A 72-year-old retired English professor with a long history of hypertension has been having difficulties with tasks he used to find easy and enjoyable, such as crossword puzzles and letter writing, because he cannot remember the correct words and his handwriting has deteriorated. He has also been having difficulties remembering the events of previous days and he moves and thinks at a slower pace. Subsequently, he develops slurred speech. Which of the following diagnoses is most likely in this patient?

a. Multi-infarct dementia
b. German-Strausser syndrome
c. Rett's disorder
d. Wernicke-Korsakoff syndrome
e. Alzheimer's disease

168. A previously healthy 60-year-old man undergoes a corneal transplant. Three months later, he is profoundly demented, demonstrates myoclonic jerks on exam, and has an EEG that shows periodic bursts of electrical activity superimposed on a slow background. Which of the following is this patient's most likely diagnosis?
a. Wilson's disease
b. Multi-infarct dementia
c. Creutzfeltd-Jakob disease
d. Epilepsy
e. Pseudodementia

169. A previously healthy 24-year-old woman has become irritable, moody, and unreliable. She has difficulty remembering words and facts that she used to know well. In the past month she has developed choreoathetoid movements in her upper extremities and has become clumsy. A slit-lamp examination of her eyes shows a greenish corneal ring around her irises. Which of the following is this patient's most likely diagnosis?
a. Wilson's disease
b. Pseudodementia
c. Gerstmann-Straussler syndrome
d. Rett's disorder
e. Huntington's disease

Items 170-171

170. A 22-year-old college student comes to the physician with the complaint of shortness of breath during anxiety-provoking situations, such as exams. She also notes perioral tingling, carpopedal spasms, and feelings of derealization at the same time. All of the symptoms pass after the anxiety over the situation has faded. The episodes have never occurred "out of the blue." Which of the following is the most likely diagnosis?
a. Panic disorder
b. Generalized anxiety disorder
c. Hyperventilation
d. Anxiety disorder not otherwise specified
e. Anxiety disorder secondary to a general medical condition

98 Psychiatry

171. Which of the following treatments should the physician suggest first?
a. Alprazolam prn
b. Fluoxetine daily
c. Rebreathe into a paper bag during the episode
d. Biofeedback
e. Hypnosis

172. A 25-year-old woman is brought to the physician by her boyfriend after he noticed a change in her personality over the preceding 6 months. He states that she often becomes excessively preoccupied with a single theme, often religious in nature. She was not previously a religious person. He notes that she often perseverates on a theme while she is speaking as well, and is overinclusive in her descriptions. Finally, he notes that while previously the two had a satisfying sexual life, now the patient appears to have no sex drive whatsoever. The physician finds the patient to be very emotionally intense as well. Physical examination was normal. Which of the following diagnoses is most likely?
a. Wernicke-Korsakoff syndrome
b. Temporal lobe epilepsy
c. Pick's disease
d. Multiple sclerosis
e. HIV-related dementia

173. A 23-year-old man comes to the physician with the complaint that his memory has worsened over the past 2 months and that he has difficulty concentrating. He has lost interest in his friends and his work. He has difficulty with abstract thoughts and problem solving. He has also felt depressed. MRI scan shows parenchymal abnormalities. Which of the following diagnoses is most likely?
a. Alzheimer's disease
b. Vascular dementia
c. HIV-related dementia
d. Lewy body disease
e. Binswanger's disease

Items 174–175

174. A 37-year-old alcoholic is brought to the emergency room after he was found unconscious in the street. He is hospitalized for dehydration and pneumonia. While being treated, he becomes acutely confused and agitated. He cannot move his eyes upward or to the right, and he is ataxic. Which of the following diagnoses is most likely?

a. Alcohol intoxication
b. Korsakoff's syndrome
c. Alcohol delirium
d. Wernicke's encephalopathy
e. Alcohol seizures

175. Which of the following treatments should be instituted?

a. Dilantin
b. Valium
c. Haloperidol
d. Amobarbitol
e. Thiamine

176. A 65-year-old woman is brought to the physician because she has become easily distractible, apathetic, and unconcerned about her appearance. She has trouble with remembering familiar words and locations, and she has become incontinent of urine. On physical examination, her gait is seen to be ataxic. While copying a complex picture, she makes many mistakes. The patient most likely has which of the following disorders?

a. Parkinson's disease
b. Thiamine deficiency
c. Vitamin B_{12} deficiency
d. Wilson's disease
e. Normal-pressure hydrocephalus

Items 177–179

177. A 43-year-old woman comes to the emergency room with a temperature of 101°F and a large suppurating ulcer on her left shoulder. This is the third such episode for this woman. Her physical exam is otherwise normal, other than the presence of multiple scars on her abdomen. The woman is admitted to the hospital and is observed to be holding her thermometer next to the light bulb to heat it up. When confronted, she angrily denies any such behavior and signs out of the hospital against medical advice. The patient most likely has which of the following diagnoses?

a. Malingering
b. Somatoform disorder
c. Borderline personality disorder
d. Factitious disorder
e. Body dysmorphic disorder

178. Which of the following etiologies is most likely underlying this behavior?

a. Primary gain
b. Secondary gain
c. Psychosis
d. Marginal intellectual function
e. Drug-seeking behavior

179. A 26-year-old man comes to the emergency room with the chief complaint of suicidal ideation. He is admitted into the psychiatric ward, where he is noncompliant with all treatment regimens and does not show any psychiatric symptoms other than his insistence that he is suicidal. It is subsequently discovered that he is wanted by the police, who have a warrant for his arrest. Which of the following best describes this behavior?

a. Primary gain
b. Secondary gain
c. Displacement
d. Rationalization
e. Marginal intellectual function

Items 180–181

180. A 32-year-old woman who has a chronic psychiatric disorder, multiple medical problems, and alcoholism comes to the physician because her breasts have started leaking a whitish fluid. What is the most likely cause of this symptom?

a. Haloperidol
b. Oral contraceptives
c. Hypothyroidism
d. Cirrhosis
e. Pregnancy

181. Which of the following endogenous substances is likely to have caused this phenomenon?

a. Estrogen
b. Thyroid hormone
c. Progesterone
d. Prolactin
e. Alcohol dehydrogenase

182. A 3-year-old child is brought to the emergency room by his parents after they found him having a generalized seizure at home. The child's breath smells of garlic, and he has bloody diarrhea, vomiting, and muscle twitching. Which of the following poisons is it likely that this child has encountered?

a. Thallium
b. Lead
c. Arsenic
d. Carbon monoxide
e. Aluminum

183. A 34-year-old woman comes to the physician with the chief complaint of pain in her neck and back. She states that 7 months previously she had been in a car accident in which she was hit from behind by a man who was angry that she wasn't traveling fast enough. Immediately after the accident the man got out of the car and began screaming at the patient. The patient had been taken to the hospital, and an exam showed severe bruising and muscular rigidity of her back and neck, but no other damage. However, the patient states she has been completely disabled by her pain since that time. She states that her life would be perfect without the pain, and pleads with the physician to make it stop. On physical exam, she has mild muscular tension in her neck and back, but otherwise her diagnostic workup is within normal limits. Which of the following diagnoses is most likely?

a. Pain disorder
b. Malingering
c. Factitious disorder
d. Hypochondriasis
e. Conversion disorder

184. Which of the following statements is true about factitious disorder?

a. It is seen more frequently in women over the age of 65
b. It is present in less than 0.5% of patients admitted to a hospital
c. The prognosis is excellent with behavioral treatment
d. The patient is primarily motivated by financial gain
e. It has been termed Munchausen syndrome

185. A man given a sugar pill for mild pain reports that 15 min later the pain has completely resolved. Which of the following conclusions is most appropriate to this occurrence?

a. The man is drug seeking
b. The man is malingering
c. The man has a factitious disorder
d. The man is demonstrating a placebo response
e. The man had no real pain to begin with

186. A 53-year-old woman has consumed over 1 pint of bourbon per day for the past 24 years. She presents with severe cognitive deficits and is diagnosed with Korsakoff's syndrome. Which of the following is she most likely to display on mental status exam?
a. Impaired recent memory and anterograde amnesia
b. Hypermnesia
c. Both anterograde and retrograde memory deficits
d. Retrograde amnesia
e. Retrospective falsification

187. A 55-year-old man comes to the physician with the chief complaint of weight loss and a depressed mood. He feels tired all the time and is no longer interested in the normal activities he previously enjoyed. He feels quite apathetic overall. He has also noticed that he has frequent, nonspecific abdominal pain. Which of the following diagnoses needs to be ruled out in this man?
a. Pheochromocytoma
b. Pancreatic carcinoma
c. Adrenocortical insufficiency
d. Cushing's syndrome
e. Huntington's disease

188. A 15-year-old girl develops generalized tonic-clonic seizures after a brain injury. She is started on valproic acid and is well controlled for the next 3 years. She leaves for college at 18, and the seizures are noted to increase in frequency dramatically, though her valproate levels remain therapeutic. If administered within 20 min after one of these episodes, which of the following tests may help in the differential diagnosis of seizure vs. pseudoseizure?
a. Prolactin level
b. Calcium level
c. TSH level
d. Cortisol level
e. Electromyography

189. Which of the following is the most common cause of delirium in the elderly?
a. Substance abuse
b. Accidental poisoning
c. Hypoxia
d. Use of multiple medications
e. Alcohol withdrawal

190. A 35-year-old woman comes to the physician with the chief complaint of recurrent episodes of irritability, dysphoria, and fatigue that occur on a monthly basis. Which of the following statements is correct about this condition?
a. The symptoms of this condition will end at menopause
b. Less than 10% of women of childbearing age complain of these symptoms
c. The symptoms reach a maximum of intensity about 5 days before the menstrual period begins
d. Excessive exposure to endogenous aldosterone may contribute to this disorder
e. The disorder has a purely psychological etiology

191. A 52-year-old man undergoes a successful mitral valve replacement. He is sent to the intensive care unit to recover. The day after the surgery, he appears irritable and restless. Hours later he is agitated, disoriented, hypervigilant, and uncooperative. This agitation alternates with periods of somnolence. Which of the following is most likely to be helpful?
a. Intramuscular Thorazine
b. Oral alprazolam
c. Modification of environment
d. Oral lithium
e. Supportive psychotherapy

192. A 23-year-old woman comes to the physician with the chief complaint of a depressed mood for 6 months. She states that she has felt lethargic, does not sleep well, and has decreased energy and difficulty concentrating. She notes that she has gained over 15 lb without attempting to do so, and seems to bruise much more easily than previously. On physical exam, she is noted to have numerous purple striae on her abdomen, proximal muscle weakness, and a loss of peripheral vision. A brain tumor is found on MRI. In which of the following areas of the brain is this tumor most likely found?
a. Frontal lobe
b. Cerebellum
c. Thalamus
d. Pituitary
e. Brainstem

193. A 34-year-old man comes to the physician with the chief complaint of new onset visual hallucinations for 1 month. He states that he sees flashing lights and movement when he knows that there is no one in the room with him. He also complains of a headache that occurs several times per week and is dull and achy in nature. He is noted on physical examination to have papilledema and a homonymous hemianopsia. A brain tumor is found on MRI. In which of the following areas of the brain is this tumor most likely found?
a. Frontal lobe
b. Parietal lobe
c. Occipital lobe
d. Temporal lobe
e. Cerebellum

194. A 26-year-old man comes to the physician with the chief complaint that he has been uncharacteristically moody and irritable. On several occasions his wife has noted that he has had angry outbursts at the children, so severe that she had to step in between him and them. He states that he has "spells" in which he smells the odors of rotten eggs and burning rubber. During this time he feels disconnected from his surroundings, as if he were in a dream. A brain tumor is found on MRI. In which of the following areas of the brain is this tumor most likely found?

a. Frontal lobe
b. Parietal lobe
c. Occipital lobe
d. Temporal lobe
e. Cerebellum

195. A 43-year-old man comes to the physician with the chief complaint of nervousness and excitability for 3 months. He states that he feels this way constantly, and this is a dramatic change for his normally relaxed personality. He notes that on occasion he becomes extremely afraid of his own impending death, even when there is no objective evidence that this would occur. He notes that he has lost 20 lb and frequently has diarrhea. On mental status examination, he is noted to have pressured speech. On physical examination, he is noted to have a fine tremor and tachycardia. Which of the following disorders is this patient most likely to have?

a. Hyperthyroidism
b. Hypothyroidism
c. Hepatic encephalopathy
d. Hyperparathyroidism
e. Hypoparathyroidism

DIRECTIONS: Each group of questions below consists of lettered options followed by a set of numbered items. For each numbered item, select the **one** lettered option with which it is **most** closely associated. Each lettered option may be used once, more than once, or not at all.

Items 196–200

Match each disorder with the most appropriate diagnostic test.
a. Hematocrit
b. Prolactin
c. Vitamin B_{12}
d. Creatinine phosphokinase (CPK)
e. ECG
f. Urine copper
g. Urine VMA
h. VDRL
i. Serum ammonia

196. Nonepileptic seizures **(CHOOSE 1 TEST)**

197. Neuroleptic malignant syndrome **(CHOOSE 1 TEST)**

198. Hepatic encephalopathy **(CHOOSE 1 TEST)**

199. Tertiary syphilis **(CHOOSE 1 TEST)**

200. Pheochromocytoma **(CHOOSE 1 TEST)**

201. A 28-year-old woman comes to the physician requesting genetic counseling. Her father has been diagnosed with Huntington's disease. What is this woman's risk for developing this disease?
a. 1 in 2
b. 1 in 4
c. 1 in 16
d. 1 in 32
e. She will not develop the disease, but will be a carrier

202. Which of the following is the most common cause of dementia?

a. Major depression
b. Alzheimer's disease
c. Normal-pressure hydrocephalus
d. Vitamin B_{12} deficiency
e. Multiple small infarcts

203. An 8-year-old boy is brought to the emergency room after being hit on the head by a baseball. His father tells the physician that after a brief period of unconsciousness, the boy quickly woke up and was alert and oriented after the incident. Shortly after the boy arrives in the emergency room, he begins complaining of a severe headache and becomes alternately somnolent and agitated as well as disoriented. On examination, he is noted to have a cranial nerve palsy as well. Which of the following is the most likely diagnosis?

a. Subdural hematoma
b. Epidural bleeding
c. Conversion disorder
d. Subarachnoid hemorrhage
e. Concussion

204. A 56-year-old retired boxer is brought to the physician by his wife because his memory is "not what it used to be." On examination, he is noted to have a moderately severe cognitive impairment. He shows little facial expression and he walks with small, rigid steps. Which of the following is the most likely cause for his disorder?

a. An idiopathic degenerative process
b. Chronic trauma
c. An inborn error of metabolism
d. A familial disorder
e. A vitamin deficiency

Cognitive Disorders and Consultation-Liaison Psychiatry

Answers

151. The answer is d. *(Ebert, p 205.)* Alzheimer's disease is the most common dementing disorder in North America, Europe, and Scandinavia. Typical symptoms are progressive memory loss, aphasia, anomia (inability to recall the name of objects), apraxia (inability to perform voluntary motor activity in the absence of motor and sensory deficits), and agnosia (inability to process and understand sensory stimuli in the absence of sensory deficits). Motor functions are spared until the very end. Personality is preserved in the early stages of the disorder, but considerable deterioration follows in later stages.

152. The answer is b. *(Kaplan, 8/e, pp 1294–1295.)* Pick's disease accounts for 2.5% of cases of dementia. Clinically it is distinguishable from Alzheimer's disease due to the prominence and early onset of personality changes, disinhibition or apathy, socially inappropriate behavior, mood changes (elation or depression), and psychotic symptoms. Language is affected early in the disease, but the memory loss, apraxia, and agnosia characteristic of Alzheimer's disease are not prominent until the late stages of the disorder. Temporofrontal atrophy, demyelination and gliosis of the frontal lobes, Pick bodies (intracellular inclusions), and Pick cells (swollen neurons) are the characteristic pathological findings.

153. The answer is e. *(Kaplan, 8/e, p 518.)* The agitation, hypervigilance, and anxiety that this man presents with are common in cocaine-intoxicated states. The man in the question gives a history that nothing like this has ever happened before, and he is a young graduate student, making Pick's disease unlikely. Similarly, the lack of any obvious other medical condition in a previously healthy patient makes delirium unlikely. Vitamin B_{12} deficiency would not have presented with these signs and symptoms, nor would dissociative disorder.

154. The answer is c. *(Kaplan, 8/e, p 721.)* Anorexia nervosa is characterized by the refusal to maintain a minimal normal weight for height and age, intense fear of gaining weight, distorted body image, and amenorrhea. Body weight is controlled by drastic reduction of caloric intake, but most anorectic patients also use diuretics and laxatives. Purging, which causes hypokalemic alkalosis, can also be present but is not as frequent as in bulimia. The other listed behaviors are not characteristic of patients with anorexia.

155. The answer is a. *(Kaplan, 8/e, p 269.)* Chronic subdural hematoma causes a reversible form of dementia. It frequently follows head trauma (60% of the cases) with tearing of the bridging veins in the subdural space. Ruptured aneurysms, rapid deceleration injuries, and arterovenous malformations (AVMs) of the pial surface account for the nontraumatic cases. The most common symptoms of chronic subdural hematomas are headache, confusion, inattention, apathy, memory loss, drowsiness, and coma. Lateralization signs, such as hemiparesis, hemianopsia, and cranial nerve abnormalities, are less prominent features. Epidural hematoma usually follows a temporal or parietal skull fracture that causes the laceration of the middle meningeal artery or vein. It is characterized by a brief period of lucidity followed by loss of consciousness, hemiparesis, cranial nerve palsies, and death unless the hematoma is surgically evacuated. Multi-infarct dementia and Alzheimer's disease are characterized by a slower onset and have a more chronic course, although diagnostic confusion is possible at times. Korsakoff's disorder is characterized by anterograde and retrograde memory deficits. Frontal lobe tumors mainly present with personality and behavioral changes, which differ depending on the localization.

156. The answer is a. *(Kaplan, 8/e, p 630.)* A conversion disorder usually presents in a monosymptomatic manner, acutely, and simulating a physical disease. The sensory or motor symptoms present are not fully explained by any known pathophysiology. The diagnostic features are such that the physical symptom is incompatible with known physiological mechanisms or anatomy. Usually an unconscious psychological stress or conflict is present. In hypochondriasis, a patient is overly concerned that he or she has an illness or illnesses; this conviction can temporarily be appeased by physician reassurance, but the reassurance generally does not last long. Factitious disorder usually presents with physical or mental symptoms that are induced by the patient to meet the psychological need to be taken care of (primary gain). Malingering is similar to factitious disorder in that symptoms are faked, but the reason in malingering is for some secondary gain, such as getting out of jail. In delusional disorder with somatic delusions, the patient has an unshakable belief that he or she has some physical defect or a medical condition.

157. The answer is c. *(Kaplan, 8/e, p 1123.)* Psychiatric symptoms are common in patients with Parkinson's disease. Affective disorders are particularly frequent, with an incidence estimated between 20 and 90%. Among affective disorders, depression and dysthymic disorder are the most frequent types. Psychotic disorders have a lower incidence (12% in one study). They are usually caused by anticholinergic and dopaminergic drug side effects, although psychosis similar to schizophrenia has been reported in the absence of medication side effects.

158. The answer is e. *(Kaplan, 8/e, p 281.)* In partial complex seizures, an altered state of consciousness, usually manifested by staring, is accompanied by hallucinations (olfactory hallucinations are common), automatisms (buttoning and unbuttoning, masticatory movements, speech automatisms), perceptual alterations (objects changing shape or size), complex verbalizations, and autonomic symptoms such as piloerection, gastric sensation, or nausea. Flashbacks, déjà vu, and derealization are also common. The episodes last approximately 1 min, and patients may experience postictal headaches and sleepiness. Absence seizure episodes are shorter, are not accompanied by motor activity, and are not followed by postictal phenomena.

159. The answer is a. *(Ebert, p 441.)* Sleep apnea is the cessation of breathing during sleep for 10 s or more. In obstructive sleep apnea, breathing stops due to airway blockage, while in central sleep apnea the breathing stops due to an absence of respiratory efforts secondary to a neurological dysfunction. Features associated with obstructive sleep apnea are excessive daytime somnolence, snoring, restless sleep, and nocturnal awakening with gasping for air. Patients often wake up in the morning with dry mouth and headache. Predisposing factors are maleness, middle age, obesity, hypothyroidism, and various malformations of the upper airways. Narcolepsy is characterized by irresistible urges to fall asleep for brief periods during the day, regardless of the situation. Nocturnal myoclonus refers to stereotyped, repetitive movements of the legs during sleep, accompanied by brief arousal and sleep disruption.

160. The answer is b. (*Kaplan, 8/e, p 66.*) Elisabeth Kübler-Ross postulated that dying patients go through five stages from the first moment they are aware of their fatal condition to the day of their death. The first stage is denial, and, if it does not interfere with treatment, it can be helpful for mitigating the initial overwhelming anxiety. In the second stage, anger toward themselves, caretakers, family, and God predominates. The third stage is bargaining for more time, most commonly by promising to change for the better if life is prolonged. When the patient arrives at the full realization of impending death, he or she enters the stage of depression. In the final stage of acceptance, the patient has accepted the inevitability of death without despair. These five stages do not represent a rigid evolutive process. Many patients fluctuate from one stage to another or go through only two or three stages. Other patients exhibit different coping styles such as the use of humor or compassion.

161. The answer is c. (*Kaplan, 8/e, p 786.*) Patients with borderline personalities see others (and themselves) as wholly good or totally bad, a psychological defense called splitting. They alternatively idealize or devalue important figures in their lives, depending on their perceptions of the others' intentions, interest, and level of caring. These dynamics often elicit similar responses in the environment, with the individuals being idealized having a considerably better opinion of the patient than those who are being devalued.

162. The answer is c. (*Kaplan, 8/e, p 820.*) Cushing's syndrome due to exogenous administration of corticosteroids and more rarely to adrenocarcinoma or ectopic production of ACTH is often associated with psychiatric disturbances. Depression and mixed anxiety and depressive states are the most common psychiatric manifestations of the syndrome (from 35 to 68%, depending on the study). Since the affective symptoms are directly secondary to the administration of a substance (in this case steroids for the treatment of asthma), the patient's diagnosis would be a substance-induced mood disorder. Mania, psychosis, delirium, and cognitive disturbances also occur, but at a much lower rate. Depressive symptoms occur early in

Cognitive Disorders and Consultation-Liaison Psychiatry   Answers   113

the disorder (in the prodromal period in 27% of cases). Most patients improve after the primary disorder is treated and serum cortisol decreases.

163. The answer is b. *(Kaplan, 8/e, p 820.)* Two or more distinct episodes of neurological impairment that cannot be explained by a single CNS lesion and multiple areas of white matter demyelination (seen as areas of hyperdensity on the MRI) are characteristic of multiple sclerosis (MS). Psychiatric disturbances (mostly depression) and cognitive impairment are frequent manifestations of this disease. The prevalence rates of depression in patients with MS range from 45 to 62%. The mood disorder secondary to a general medical condition appears to be a direct consequence of the brain demyelination more than a psychological reaction to living with a chronic disease. Attention, memory, and problem-solving deficits are also frequent in MS.

164. The answer is d. *(Kaplan, 8/e, p 281.)* Hallucinations involving smell, taste, or kinesthetic experiences (body movements) are rare. They are most commonly encountered in patients with partial complex seizures, although occasionally they are reported by patients with somatization disorder, psychosis, or hypochondriasis. Tumors involving the olfactory areas of the brain must also be considered in the differential diagnosis.

165. The answer is c. *(Kaplan, 8/e, p 821.)* Huntington's disease is a neurodegenerative disorder characterized by choreic movements of the face, limbs, and trunk; progressive dementia; and psychiatric symptoms. Deficits in sustained attention, memory retrieval, procedural memory (ability to acquire new skills), and visuospatial skills are predominant and early manifestations of the disorder. Language skills are usually preserved until the late stages of the disease. Personality changes and mood disturbances, including depression and mania, are frequent and can predate the onset of the dementia and the movement disorder. Neuroimaging reveals atrophy of the caudate and the putamen.

166. The answer is c. *(Kaplan, 8/e, p 821.)* Impaired naming, memory deterioration, poor calculation, poor judgment, and disinhibition are characteristic symptoms of Alzheimer's disease. This progressive dementia develops in all individuals with trisomy 21 (Down syndrome) who survive beyond 30 years. Neurofibrillary tangles, neuritic plaques, and loss of acetylcholine neurons in the nucleus basalis of Meynert—characteristic pathological changes of Alzheimer's disease—develop in patients with Down syndrome at a relatively young adult age.

167. The answer is a. *(Kaplan, 8/e, p 821.)* Multi-infarct dementia results from the cumulative effects of multiple small- and large-vessel occlusions in cortical and subcortical regions. Most cases are caused by hypertensive cerebrovascular disease and thrombo-occlusive disease. It is the second most common cause of dementia in the elderly, accounting for 8 to 35% of the cases. Clinically, it is characterized by memory and cognitive deficits accompanied by focal neurologic signs (muscle weakness, spasticity, dysarthria, extensor plantar reflex, etc.). Unlike Alzheimer's disease, multi-infarct dementia is characterized by sudden onset and a stepwise progression.

168. The answer is c. *(Ebert, p 222.)* Creutzfeldt-Jakob disease is a neurodegenerative disease caused by a transmissible infectious agent, the prion. Most cases are iatrogenic, following transplant of infected corneas or use of contaminated neurosurgical instruments. Familial forms, following an autosomal dominant pattern of inheritance, represent 5 to 15% of cases. Patients show a very rapid cognitive deterioration, myoclonic jerks, rigidity, and ataxia. Death follows within a year. An intermittent periodic burst pattern (periodic complexes) is the characteristic EEG finding. Epilepsy causes spike and wave patterns on EEG, and may cause postseizure memory loss and disorientation (in generalized, tonic-clonic seizures) or a depersonalization syndrome (in temporal lobe epilepsy or other focal seizure disorder), but would not be expected to cause dementia, continuous myoclonic jerks on exam, or an EEG that shows periodic bursts of electrical activity superimposed on a slow background. Pseudodementia is the term used in patients with major depression who exhibit impaired attention, perception, problem solving, or memory. The cognitive decline is often more precipitous than in demented patients. Patient history often reveals past major depressive episodes. Although the actual memory impairment is modest in these patients, the subjective complaint is high.

169. The answer is a. *(Kaplan, 8/e, p 821.)* Wilson's disease, or hepatolenticular degeneration, is an autosomal recessive disorder of copper metabolism (deficiency of the copper-carrying protein ceruloplasmin). Frequency is 1 in 40,000 births. The disease first manifests in the second or third decade with a combination of neurologic symptoms (tremor, rigidity, poor coordination, abnormalities of gait and posture), mild impairment of memory retrieval and executive functions, and, in 20% of patients, psychiatric symptoms such as personality changes and mood disturbances. Copper corneal deposits (Kayser-Fleischer rings) are present in most patients. Other diagnostic findings are chronic hepatitis, hemolytic anemia, and cavitary necrosis of the putamen. Gerstmann-Straussler syndrome is a rare familial dementia caused by a prion and is related to Creutzfeldt-Jakob syndrome. It resembles olivopontocerebellar degeneration and is accompanied by spongiform encephalopathy. Rett's disorder is a disorder of childhood in which a child with apparently normal prenatal and perinatal development suddenly experiences a deceleration of head growth before age 2, with the loss of previously acquired hand skills, social engagement, coordination, and language development.

170. The answer is c. *(Kaplan, 8/e, p 880. Ebert, p 337.)* Hyperventilation causes hypocapnia and respiratory alkalosis, which in turn lead to decreased cerebral blood flow and a decrease in ionized serum calcium. Dizziness, derealization, and light-headedness are due to the cerebral vasoconstriction, while circumoral tingling, carpopedal spasm, and paresthesias are symptoms of hypocalcemia. Hyperventilation is a central feature of panic disorder and acute anxiety attacks, though more symptoms are required (beyond just hyperventilation) to make those diagnoses. Panic disorder is characterized by recurring, spontaneous, unexpected anxiety attacks with rapid onset and short duration. The symptoms of an attack climb to maximum intensity within 10 min, but can peak within a few seconds. Typical symptoms include shortness of breath, tachypnea, tachycardia, tremor, dizziness, hot or cold sensations, chest discomfort, and feelings of depersonalization or derealization. A minimum of four symptoms is required to meet the diagnosis of panic attack. Generalized anxiety disorder is characterized by excessive anxiety and worry occurring more days than not for at least 6 months about a number of events or activities. The anxiety and worry are associated with three or more of six symptoms: (1) restlessness or feeling keyed up or on edge, (2) becoming easily fatigued, (3) difficulty concentrating, (4) irritability, (5) muscle tension, (6) sleep disturbance. Anxiety disorder not otherwise specified is characterized by similar constellations of symptoms with one of the other

DSM-IV diagnoses (panic disorder, phobia, GAD, PTSD, etc.). There are insufficient criteria to meet any one of the diagnoses, but perhaps a number of symptoms for several. Anxiety disorder secondary to a general medical condition is characterized by symptoms of anxiety, but these symptoms must be related to (and caused by) a medical illness, such as hyperthyroidism, angina, hypoglycemia, etc.

171. The answer is c. *(Kaplan, 8/e, p 880.)* Given that the diagnosis in this case is hyperventilation, the treatment of choice is rebreathing into a paper bag. In doing so, the hypocapnia is reversed, as is the respiratory alkalosis, which in turn leads to a return of normal cerebral blood flow and a normalization of the ionized serum calcium. All signs and symptoms will disappear from there. After the hyperventilation episodes are stopped, it might be advisable for the patient to learn relaxation techniques (perhaps through biofeedback or hypnosis) so that the episodes will not recur. Neither a benzodiazepine or an antidepressant is indicated in this case.

172. The answer is b. *(Kaplan, 8/e, p 93.)* Temporal lobe epilepsy may often manifest as bizarre behavior without the classic grand mal shaking movements caused by seizures in the motor cortex. A TLE personality is characterized by hyposexuality, emotional intensity, and a perseverative approach to interactions, termed viscosity. Wernicke-Korsakoff syndrome is a neurologic condition manifested by confusion, ataxia, and nystagmus; thiamine deficiency is its direct cause. If thiamine is given during the acute stage of Wernicke's encephalopathy, Korsakoff's syndrome can be prevented. This syndrome is characterized by a severe anterograde learning defect associated with confabulations. Although Wernicke-Korsakoff's can be caused by malnutrition alone, it is usually associated with alcohol abuse and dependence. Pick's disease is a form of frontal lobe dementia in which Pick's cells and bodies (irregularly shaped, silver-staining, intracytoplasmic inclusion bodies that displace the nucelus toward the periphery) are present in the brain. There is an insidious onset and gradual progression, with early decline in social interpersonal conduct. Emotional blunting and apathy also occur early without insight into them. There is a marked decline in personal hygiene and significant distractibility and motor impersistence.

173. The answer is c. *(Kaplan, 8/e, p 332.)* HIV dementia is the most frequent neurological complication of HIV infection and can be the first

Cognitive Disorders and Consultation-Liaison Psychiatry Answers

symptom of the infection. It is due to a direct effect of the virus on the brain and is always accompanied by some brain atrophy. HIV dementia presents with the combination of cognitive impairment, motor deficits, and behavioral changes typical of a subcortical dementia. Common features include impaired attention and concentration, psychomotor slowing, forgetfulness, slow reaction time, and mood changes.

174–175. The answers are 174-d, 175-e. (Kaplan, 8/e, p 878.) Wernicke's encephalopathy occurs in nutritionally deficient alcoholics and is due to thiamine deficiency and consequent damage of the thiamine-dependent brain structures, including the mammillary bodies and the dorsomedial nucleus of the thalamus. It presents with mental confusion, ataxia, and sixth nerve paralysis. Wernicke's encephalopathy is a medical emergency and can rapidly resolve with immediate supplementation of thiamine.

176. The answer is e. (Ebert, p 222.) Normal-pressure hydrocephalus (NPH) is an idiopathic disorder caused by the obstruction of the flow of the cerebrospinal fluid (CSF) into the subarachnoid space. Onset usually occurs after age 60. The classic syndrome of normal-pressure hydrocephalus consists of dementia, gait abnormality, and urinary incontinence. The dementia has frontal-subcortical dysfunction features, such as impaired attention, visuospatial deficits, and poor judgment. Apathy, inertia, and lack of concern are the typical personality changes. Ventricular dilatation without sulcal widening (that is, without evidence of atrophy) and normal CSF pressure during lumbar puncture are diagnostic. The dementia can be reversed with a CSF shunt, especially if the course of the disease is short.

177–179. The answers are 177-d, 178-a, 179-b. (Ebert, pp 378, 383.) Factitious disorder usually presents with physical or mental symptoms that are induced by the patient to meet the psychological need to be taken care of (primary gain). These patients will often mutilate themselves repeatedly in a frantic effort to be cared for by the hospital system. Moving between hospitals so that they don't get caught is frequent, especially when the patient is directly confronted. Malingering is similar to factitious disorder in that symptoms are faked, but the reason in malingering is for some secondary gain, such as getting out of jail. Somatization disorder is characterized by the recurrent physical complaints that are not explained by physical factors and that cause significant impairment or result in seeking medical attention. Pain of any part of the body and dysfunctions of multiple systems are typical. The DSM-IV diagnostic criteria for somatization disorder include at least four pain symptoms, one sexual symptom, and one pseudoneurological symptom. These symptoms can be present at any time in the duration of the disorder. Somatization disorder usually emerges in adolescence or early twenties and follows a chronic course. Somatization disorder is diagnosed predominantly in women, with a prevalence of 0.2 to 0.5%, and rarely in men. Body dysmorphic disorder is characterized by distorted beliefs about the patient's own appearance, often with delusional qualities. Borderline personality disorder patients may mutilate themselves, but the object is generally attention getting or stress relief.

180–181. The answers are 180-a, 181-d. *(Kaplan, 8/e, p 999.)* Neuroleptic medications can produce hyperprolactinemia even at very low doses and are the most common cause of galactorrhea in psychiatric patients. Hyperprolactinemia with neuroleptic use is secondary to the blockade of dopamine receptors with these drugs. (Dopamine normally inhibits prolactin, and with dopamine's blockade, hyperprolactinemia can result.) Amenorrhea and galactorrhea are the main symptoms of hyperprolactinemia in women, and impotence is the main symptom in men, although men can also develop gynecomastia and galactorrhea. Other causes of hyperprolactinemia include severe systemic illness such as cirrhosis or renal failure, pituitary tumors, idiopathic causes, and pregnancy.

182. The answer is c. *(Harrison's Online, p 13.)* Acute arsenic poisoning from ingestion results in increased permeability of small blood vessels and inflammation and necrosis of the intestinal mucosa; these changes manifest as hemorrhagic gastroenteritis, fluid loss, and hypotension. Symptoms include nausea, vomiting, diarrhea, abdominal pain, delirium, coma, and seizures. A garlicky odor may be detectable on the breath. Arsenic is found in herbal and homeopathic remedies, insecticides, rodenticides, and wood preservatives, and it has a variety of other industrial applications.

183. The answer is a. *(Kaplan, 8/e, p 642.)* Pain disorder is defined as the presence of pain that is the predominant focus of clinical attention. Psychological factors play an important role in the disorder. The primary symptom is pain, in one or more sites, that is not fully accounted for by a nonpsychiatric medical or neurological condition. The symptoms of pain are associated with emotional distress and functional impairment.

184. The answer is e. *(Kaplan, 8/e, p 656.)* Factitious disorder is described as the intentional fabrication or feigning of psychological or physical signs and symptoms with the intent to assume the sick role. The possible presentations range from total fabrication of symptoms to actual illness production (for example, by injecting fecal material under the skin to create an abscess). Many kinds of medical, surgical, or psychiatric illnesses have been reproduced or fabricated, from such common disorders as urinary tract infections to obscure entities as Goodpasture syndrome (hemoptysis and glomerulonephritis). Different motivations distinguish factitious disorder from malingering, since in the latter the patients create or simulate symptoms to avoid work or legal prosecution or to obtain financial gains. Patients with somatization disorder do not voluntarily produce or feign their symptoms, while in masochism, patients submit to pain with the intent to reach sexual gratification. A severe form of factitious disorder that involves numerous hospitalizations and moving from one medical center to another to avoid discovery is called Munchhausen syndrome. Patients with Munchhausen syndrome are usually middle-aged men, unmarried, unemployed, and estranged from their families. Women between the ages of 20 and 40 represent the majority of patients with a less dramatic presentation of the disorder. Factitious disorder is not rare, but, because it is difficult to diagnose due to the patients' deception and their tendency to change doctors and hospitals, its incidence is not well known. Rates range from 0.3% of neurological disorders treated at a Berlin hospital to 9.3% of all cases of fever of unknown origin reviewed by the National Institute for Allergies and Infectious Diseases.

185. The answer is d. *(Kaplan, 8/e, p 1126.)* A placebo is an inactive substance disguised as an active treatment. It can be effective in pain with both psychogenic and organic causes. Consequently, the only conclusion that can be reached about the man described in the question is that he responds to placebos. His response says nothing about whether his pain is real or psychogenic. Many psychological factors are thought to contribute to the effects of placebos, including the patient's expectations, the provider's attitude toward the patient and the treatment, and conditioned responses.

186. The answer is a. *(Kaplan, 8/e, p 402.)* Korsakoff's psychosis is characterized by both anterograde and retrograde memory deficits. Patients cannot form new memories, and they have difficulties recalling past personal events, with the poorest recall for events that took place closest to the onset of the amnesia. Remote memories are usually preserved.

187. The answer is b. *(Kaplan, 8/e, p 820.)* Pancreatic carcinoma should always be considered in depressed middle-aged patients. It presents with weight loss, abdominal pain, apathy, decreased energy, lethargy, anhedonia, and depression. An elevated amylase can sometimes be found in laboratory testing. The other disorders listed do not present in this manner.

188. The answer is a. *(Kaplan, 8/e, p 635.)* After a generalized tonic-clonic seizure, prolactin levels increase dramatically, but they remain at baseline values in nonepileptic seizures. Blood samples must be drawn within 20 min of the episode. This test is less reliable with partial complex seizures, and it is not useful in status epilepticus and simple partial seizures.

189. The answer is d. *(Ebert, p 199.)* The use of multiple medications (polypharmacy) is among the most common causes of delirium in elderly patients, especially patients who already have signs of cognitive deterioration and many medical problems. Drug abuse and drug withdrawal are more commonly seen in young and middle-aged adults. Accidental poisoning and hypoxia (for example, from drowning) are more frequent in children.

190. The answer is c. *(Kaplan, 8/e, pp 808–809.)* Premenstrual dysphoric disorder and premenstrual syndrome are characterized by cyclical subjective changes in the mood and general sense of physical and psychological well-being correlated with the menstrual cycle. The symptoms usually begin soon after ovulation, increase gradually, and reach a maximum of intensity about 5 days before the menstrual period begins. Premenstrual dysphoric disorder and PMS also occur in women past menopause and after hysterectomy, as long as the ovaries remain intact. Seventy to 90 percent of all women of childbearing age report at least some symptoms. Psychological, social, and biological factors have been implicated in the disorder's pathogenesis. In particular, changes in estrogen, progesterone, androgen, and prolactin levels have been hypothesized to be important.

Cognitive Disorders and Consultation-Liaison Psychiatry   Answers

191. The answer is c. *(Kaplan, 8/e, p 823.)* Postcardiotomy delirium is a frequent complication of cardiac surgery, with a prevalence that has remained constant through the years at 32%. Drugs effects, especially from opioids and anticholinergic medications; subclinical brain injury; complement activation; poor nutritional status; and embolism have been among the identified causes of this syndrome. Stable vital signs help in the differential diagnosis with delirium tremens, which is accompanied by hypertension, tachycardia, and elevated temperature. The addition of medications on top of this picture usually does not help, and may worsen the condition. (If medications are necessary to control agitation, a small dose of a high-potency neuroleptic is the treatment of choice.) Frequent orientation of the patient to his or her surroundings and the personnel there usually helps.

192. The answer is d. *(Kaplan, 8/e, p 820.)* Tumors of the pituitary cause bitemporal hemianopsia by compressing the optic chiasm and a variety of endocrine disturbances that in turn can cause psychiatric symptoms. The woman in the question has a basophilic adenoma, and her depression is part of her Cushing's syndrome. Patients with craniopharyngiomas can also present with behavioral and autonomic disturbances caused by the upward extension of the tumor into the diencephalon.

193. The answer is c. *(Kaplan, 8/e, p 819.)* Occipital lobe tumors present with headache, papilledema, and homonymous hemianopsia. Visual problems and seizures are common. Patients may also complain of visual hallucinations or auras of flashing lights and movement.

194. The answer is d. *(Kaplan, 8/e, p 819.)* Tumors of the temporal lobe can present with olfactory and other unusual types of hallucinations, derealization episodes, mood lability, irritability, intermittent anger, and behavioral dyscontrol. Anxiety is another frequent finding.

195. The answer is a. *(Kaplan, 8/e, p 819.)* Patients with hyperthyroidism complain of heat intolerance and excessive sweating, as well as diarrhea, weight loss, tachycardia, palpitations, and vomiting. Psychiatric complaints can include nervousness, excitability, irritability, pressured speech, insomnia, psychosis, and a fear of impending death or doom. Decreased concentration, hyperactivity, and a fine tremor may also be found.

196–200. The answers are 196-b, 197-d, 198-i, 199-h, 200-g. *(Kaplan, 8/e, pp 264–268.)* Grand mal seizures are followed by a sharp rise in serum prolactin level that lasts approximately 20 min. Since in nonepileptic seizures prolactin levels do not change, this test may be helpful in the differential diagnosis. In neuroleptic malignant syndrome, the severe muscle contraction causes rhabdomyolysis and an increase of the serum CPK level. CPK levels also increase with dystonic reactions and following intramuscular injections. Serum ammonia is increased in delirium secondary to hepatic encephalopathy. Gastrointestinal hemorrhages and severe cardiac failure may also cause an increase in serum ammonia. A VDRL is helpful in the diagnosis of tertiary syphilis, which can present with irresponsible behavior, irritability, and confusion. A pheochromocytoma, diagnosed with a urine VMA, may present with a variety of psychiatric symptoms, including anxiety, apprehension, panic, diaphoresis, and tremor.

201. The answer is a. *(Ebert, p 211.)* Huntington's disease is an autosomal dominant disorder, and in affected families the risk for developing the disease is 50%. Huntington's disease has been traced to an area of unstable DNA on chromosome 4.

202. The answer is b. *(Kaplan, 8/e, pp 123, 328.)* The most common cause of dementia is Alzheimer's disease. Together with vascular (multi-infarct) dementia, it accounts for 75% of all cases. In the United States, approximately 5% of people older than age 65 have severe dementia and 15% have mild dementia. Of all patients with dementia, 50 to 60% have dementia of the Alzheimer's type.

203. The answer is b. *(Hales, 4/e, p 334.)* Epidural hematomas usually follow a fracture of the parietal or temporal bones and the subsequent laceration of the middle meningeal artery or vein. They are characterized by delirium and loss of consciousness that usually follow a brief period of lucidity; hemiparesis; and cranial nerve palsies. Left untreated, these hematomas are often fatal. Subdural hematomas can be spontaneous, or, more frequently, they follow a head trauma, usually within 48 h. They are caused by a tear of the bridging veins in the subdural space, and they cause a variety of neuropsychiatric symptoms such as headache, confusion, and cognitive deterioration, that often are confused with degenerative forms of dementia. Subarachnoid hemorrhages are due to bleeding aneurysms and arteriovenous malformations. They are characterized by the presence of blood in the CSF, severe sudden headaches, and signs of meningeal irritation.

204. The answer is b. *(Kaplan, 8/e, p 269.)* A persisting dementia called chronic traumatic encephalopathy occurs with multiple head traumas, even of minor entity. A classic example is dementia pugilistica or boxer's dementia. In this disorder, cognitive decline and memory deficits are characteristically accompanied by parkinsonian symptoms.

Schizophrenia and Other Psychotic Disorders

Questions

DIRECTIONS: Each item below contains a question or incomplete statement followed by suggested responses. Select the **one best** response to each question.

205. A 24-year-old man with chronic schizophrenia is brought to the emergency room after his parents found him in his bed and were unable to communicate with him. On examination, the man is confused and disoriented. He has severe muscle rigidity and a temperature of 103°F. His blood pressure is elevated, and he has a leucocytosis. Which of the following is the best first step in the pharmacologic treatment of this man?
a. Haloperidol
b. Lorazepam
c. Bromocriptine
d. Benztropine
e. Lithium

Items 206–207

206. A 54-year-old man with a chronic mental illness seems to be constantly chewing. He does not wear dentures. His tongue darts in and out of his mouth, and he occasionally smacks his lips. He also grimaces, frowns, and blinks excessively. Which of the following disorders is most likely in this patient?
a. Tourette's syndrome
b. Akathisia
c. Tardive dyskinesia
d. Parkinson's disease
e. Huntington's disease

207. A 58-year-old woman with a chronic mental disorder comes to the physician with irregular choreoathetoid movements of her hands and trunk. She states that the movements get worse under stressful conditions. Which of the following medications is most likely to have caused this disorder?

a. Fluoxetine
b. Clozapine
c. Perphenazine
d. Diazepam
e. Phenobarbitol

208. A 41-year-old man has been treated with haloperidol for his schizophrenia for the past 15 years. He begins to notice subtle involuntary movements of his hands, feet, lips, and tongue. Because he had been stable for over 1 year, his physician decided to decrease the patient's medication. Which of the following should the physician tell the patient about the movement disorder?

a. It will disappear as soon as the medication is decreased
b. It will increase initially as the medication is decreased
c. It will remain unchanged
d. It will disappear in his hands but not his feet as soon as the medication is decreased
e. It will disappear only if the medication can be completely discontinued

209. A 17-year-old boy is diagnosed with schizophrenia. What is the risk that one of his siblings will develop the disease?

a. 2%
b. 5%
c. 10%
d. 20%
e. 30%

210. A 24-year-old woman comes to the emergency room with the chief complaint that "my stomach is rotting out from the inside." She states that for the last 6 months she has been crying on a daily basis and that she has decreased concentration, energy, and interest in her usual hobbies. She has lost 25 lb during that time. She cannot get to sleep, and when she does, she wakes up early in the morning. For the past 3 weeks, she has become convinced that she is dying of cancer and is rotting on the inside of her body. She has also heard a voice calling her name in the past 2 weeks when no one is around. Which of the following is the most appropriate diagnosis for this patient?
a. Delusional disorder
b. Schizoaffective disorder
c. Schizophreniform disorder
d. Schizophrenia
e. Major depression with psychotic features

211. A 19-year-old man is brought to the physician by his parents after he called them from college, terrified that the Mafia was after him. He states he has eaten nothing for the past 6 weeks other than canned beans because "they are into everything—I can't be too careful." He is convinced that the Mafia has put cameras in his dormitory room and that they are watching his every move. He occasionally hears the voices of two men talking about him when no one is around. His roommate states that for the past 2 months the patient has been increasingly withdrawn and suspicious. Which of the following is the most likely diagnosis for this patient?
a. Delusional disorder
b. Schizoaffective disorder
c. Schizophreniform disorder
d. Schizophrenia
e. PCP intoxication

212. A 36-year-old woman is brought to the psychiatrist by her husband because for the past 8 months she refuses to go out of the house because she states that the neighbors are trying to harm her. She is afraid that if they see her they will hurt her, and finds many small bits of evidence supporting this fact. This evidence includes the fact that the neighbors leave their garbage cans out on the street to try to trip her, they park their cars in their driveways so that they can hide behind them and spy on her, and they walk by her house to try to get a look into where she is hiding. She states that her mood is fine, and would be "better if they would leave me alone." She denies hearing the neighbors or anyone else talk to her, but is sure that they are out to "cause her death and mayhem." Which of the following diagnoses is the most likely in this patient?

a. Delusional disorder
b. Schizophreniform disorder
c. Schizoaffective disorder
d. Schizophrenia
e. Major depression with psychotic features

213. A 35-year-old woman has lived in a state psychiatric hospital for the past 10 years. She spends most of her day rocking, muttering softly to herself, or looking at her reflection in a small mirror. She needs help with dressing and showering, and she often giggles and laughs for no apparent reason. Which of the following diagnoses is the most likely in this patient?

a. Schizophrenia, paranoid type
b. Schizophrenia, disorganized type
c. Schizophrenia, residual type
d. Schizoaffective disorder
e. Schizophreniform disorder

214. A 20-year-old woman is brought to the emergency room by her family after they were unable to get her to eat or drink anything for the past 2 days. The patient, although awake, is completely unresponsive both vocally and nonverbally. She actively resists any attempt to be moved. Her family states that for the previous 7 months she has become increasingly withdrawn, socially isolated, and bizarre, often speaking to people no one else could see. Which of the following diagnoses is the most likely in this patient?
a. Schizoaffective disorder
b. Delusional disorder
c. Schizophreniform disorder
d. Catatonia
e. PCP intoxication

215. A 21-year-old man is brought to the emergency room by his parents because he has not slept, bathed, or eaten in the past 3 days. The parents state that for the past 6 months their son has been acting strangely and "not himself." They state that he has been locking himself in his room, talking to himself, and writing on the walls. Six weeks prior to the emergency room visit, their son became convinced that a fellow student was stealing his thoughts and making him unable to learn his school material. In the past 2 weeks, they have noticed that the patient has become depressed and has stopped taking care of himself, including bathing, eating, and getting dressed. On exam, the patient is dirty, disheveled, and crying. He complains of not being able to concentrate, a low energy level, and feeling suicidal. Which of the following diagnoses is the most likely in this patient?
a. Schizoaffective disorder
b. Schizophrenia
c. Bipolar I disorder
d. Schizoid personality disorder
e. Delusional disorder

216. Which of the following statements regarding formal thought disorder is true?
a. It is found only in schizophrenia
b. It may be found in bipolar patients
c. Delusions are a form of thought disorder
d. Ideas of reference are a form of thought disorder
e. Obsessions are a form of thought disorder

130 Psychiatry

217. An otherwise healthy 45-year-old schizophrenic comes to his psychiatrist for a routine visit. He has had a poor response to several trials of typical antipsychotics, as well as risperidone and olanzepine. His psychiatrist recommends a trial of clozapine. Which of the following baseline tests should be ordered on this patient before starting this drug?
a. EEG
b. Thyroid function tests
c. Liver function tests
d. WBC count
e. BUN

218. A 47-year-old woman is brought to the emergency room after she jumped off an overpass and broke both her legs. In the emergency room she states that she wanted to kill herself because the devil had been tormenting her for many years. She becomes fearful in the emergency room as well, thinking that the devil has possessed the nursing staff working there. After stabilization of her fractures, she is admitted to the psychiatric unit, where she is treated with risperidone and sertraline. After 2 weeks she is no longer suicidal and her mood is euthymic. However, she still believes that the devil is recruiting people to try to persecute her. The patient has had 3 similar episodes prior to this one in the past 10 years. During each of these three episodes, she has been suicidal and anhedonic and has had low energy levels. During these times she also has early morning awakening, is unable to concentrate, and loses 5 to 10 lb because she has no appetite. She has never stopped believing that the devil is persecuting her during all this time. Which of the following is the most appropriate diagnosis for this patient?
a. Delusional disorder
b. Schizoaffective disorder
c. Schizophrenia, paranoid type
d. Schizophreniform disorder
e. Major depression with psychotic features

219. A 40-year-old woman is arrested by the police after she is found crawling through the window of a movie star's home. She states that the movie star invited her into his home because the two are secretly married and "it just wouldn't be good for his career if everyone knew." The movie star denies the two have ever met, but notes that the woman has sent him hundreds of letters over the past 2 years. The woman has never been in trouble before, and lives an otherwise isolated and unremarkable life. Which of the following diagnoses is this patient most likely to have?
a. Delusional disorder
b. Schizoaffective disorder
c. Bipolar I disorder
d. Cyclothymia
e. Schizophreniform disorder

220. A schizophrenic patient has no interest in social contacts or vocational rehabilitation. His affect is flat, and he speaks very little and spends most of his day sitting in front of the TV, unwashed and unshaven. He has some chronic delusions of persecution, but these do not impact his functioning as much as the previous symptoms. Which of the following antipsychotics would be most appropriate to use in treating this patient?
a. Molindone
b. Haloperidol decanoate
c. Chlorpromazine
d. Olanzapine
e. Perphenzaine

221. A 45-year-old woman is treated with an antipsychotic medication for 2 years. She develops an uneven pigmentation over her face, shoulders, and arms after a trip to the beach. Which of the following antipsychotics is she most likely taking?
a. Clozapine
b. Molindone
c. Haloperidol decanoate
d. Chlorpromazine
e. Olanzapine

222. A 55-year-old schizophrenic has been treated with haloperidol for the past 25 years. She presents with constant chewing movements, grimaces, and lip smacking. Her symptoms persist when her haloperidol dose is decreased. Without the neuroleptic, she experiences persecutory delusions and command auditory hallucinations, which tell her to kill her family members. Which of the following antipsychotics should this patient be switched to?

a. Loxitane
b. Molindone
c. Thioridazine
d. Olanzapine
e. Perphenazine

223. A schizophrenic patient has a history of multiple relapses caused by noncompliance with his antipsychotic medications. Which of the following antipsychotics should this patient be switched to?

a. Clozapine
b. Haloperidol decanoate
c. Chlorpromazine
d. Thioridazine
e. Quetiapine

224. Which of the following statements regarding delusions is true?

a. They are almost exclusively found in schizophrenia
b. Grandiose delusions are rarely encountered except in mania
c. They involve a disturbance of thought content
d. They involve a disturbance in perception
e. They are a type of hallucination

225. Approximately what percentage of schizophrenics ultimately commit suicide?

a. 1%
b. 5%
c. 10%
d. 20%
e. 30%

226. A 26-year-old woman is brought to the emergency room by her husband after she begins screaming that her children are calling to her and becomes hysterical. The husband states that 2 weeks previously the couple's two children were killed in a car accident, and since that time the patient has been agitated, disorganized, and incoherent. He states that she will not eat because she believes he has been poisoning her food, and she has not slept in the past 2 days. In the emergency room, the patient believes that the nurses are going to cause her harm as well. The patient is sedated and later sent home. One week later all her symptoms remit spontaneously. Which of the following is the most likely diagnosis for this patient?
a. Delirium
b. Schizophreniform disorder
c. Major depression with psychotic features
d. Brief psychotic disorder
e. Posttraumatic stress disorder

227. Two days after delivering a healthy, full-term baby girl, a 25-year-old woman becomes acutely agitated and disoriented. She refuses to feed her baby, stating that the baby is born of the devil. She hears voices telling her to drown her daughter if she wants to save her soul. Which of the following statements is correct?
a. The woman is having a full-blown episode of schizophrenia
b. The baby should be removed by a child protection agency immediately
c. The woman should be warned never to have another child
d. The woman's disorder is most closely related to schizophrenia
e. The woman should be treated with antipsychotic and antidepressant medications

228. Which of the following is the lifetime prevalence for schizophrenia?
a. 1%
b. 3%
c. 5%
d. 10%
e. 15%

229. A 25-year-old woman is diagnosed with schizophrenia when, after the sudden death of her mother, she begins complaining of hearing voices of the devil and is suddenly afraid that other people are out to hurt her. By history, she is also noted to have a 3-year period of slowly worsening social withdrawal, apathy, and bizarre behavior. Her family history includes major depression in her father. Which of the following details of her history leads the physician to suspect that her outcome may be poor?

a. She is female
b. She was age 25 at diagnosis
c. She had an acute precipitating factor before the appearance of hearing voices
d. She had an insidious onset to her illness
e. There is an affective disorder history in her family

230. Which of the following drugs may induce a psychosis that is easily confused with, or misdiagnosed as, paranoid schizophrenia?

a. Barbiturates
b. Heroin
c. Benzodiazepines
d. Amphetamines
e. MDMA ("ecstasy")

231. Studies of the relationship between gender and schizophrenia have generally demonstrated which of the following facts?

a. Age of onset for females is usually earlier than that for males
b. Females tend to have a worse prognosis than males
c. The impairment in male patients is, on average, greater than in female patients
d. Females respond more poorly to medication than do males
e. Female monozygotic twins have a higher concordance rate for the disease than do male monozygotic twins

232. Families of patients with schizophrenia who are overtly hostile and overly controlling affect the patient in what way?
a. Increased relapse rate
b. Decreased rate of compliance
c. High likelihood that this behavior led to the patient's first break of the disease
d. Increased likelihood that the patient's schizophrenia will be of the paranoid type
e. Decreased risk of suicidal behavior

233. A 62-year-old man with chronic schizophrenia is brought to the emergency room after he is found wandering around his halfway house confused and disoriented. His serum sodium concentration is 123 mEq/L. Urine sodium concentration is 5 mEq/L. The patient has been treated with risperidone 4 mg/d for the past 3 years with good symptom control. His roommate reports that the patient often complains of feeling thirsty. Which of the following is the most likely cause of this patient's symptoms?
a. Renal failure
b. Inappropriate antidiuretic hormone (ADH) secretion
c. Addison's disease
d. Psychogenic polydipsia
e. Nephrotic syndrome

Psychiatry

DIRECTIONS: Each group of questions below consists of lettered options followed by a set of numbered items. For each numbered item, select the **one** lettered option with which it is **most** closely associated. Each lettered option may be used once, more than once, or not at all.

Items 234–237

Match the symptoms displayed by each patient with the appropriate culture-bound syndrome.

a. Koro
b. Amok
c. Sangue dormido
d. Nervios
e. Dhat
f. Windigo
g. Mal de ojo

234. A 27-year-old man is brought to the hospital after he suddenly becomes enraged and acutely agitated. He killed several dogs that came near him during this episode. His family and friends can think of nothing that may have provoked him. The episode is self-contained, and the patient shortly returns to his previous level of functioning. **(CHOOSE 1 SYNDROME)**

235. A man is brought to the physician because he is convinced that his penis is receding into his body and that when it disappears completely, he will die. **(CHOOSE 1 SYNDROME)**

236. A Brazilian woman experiences tearfulness, inability to concentrate, headaches, dizziness, insomnia, and nervousness after her house is broken into by burglars. **(CHOOSE 1 SYNDROME)**

237. A Mediterranean man comes to the physician for symptoms including vomiting, fever, and restless sleep. He tells the physician that this was caused by someone cursing him with the evil eye. **(CHOOSE 1 SYNDROME)**

238. A 25-year-old man is brought to the physician after complaining of a visual hallucination of a transparent phantom of his own body. Which of the following specific syndromes is this patient most likely to be displaying?
a. Capgras syndrome
b. Lycanthropy
c. Cotard syndrome
d. Autoscopic psychosis
e. Folie à deux

Schizophrenia and Other Psychotic Disorders

Answers

205. The answer is c. *(Kaplan, 8/e, p 958.)* The patient has neuroleptic malignant syndrome (NMS), a life-threatening complication of antipsychotic treatment. The symptoms include muscular rigidity and dystonia, akinesia, mutism, obtundation, and agitation. The autonomic symptoms include high fever, sweating, and increased blood pressure and heart rate. Mortality rates are reported to be 10 to 20%. In addition to supportive medical treatment, the most commonly used medications for the condition are dantrolene (Dantrium) and bromocriptine (Parlodel), although amantadine is sometimes used. Bromocriptine and amantadine possess direct dopamine receptor agonist effects and may serve to overcome the antipsychotic-induced dopamine receptor blockade. Dantrolene is a direct muscle relaxant.

206. The answers are 206-c, 207-c. *(Kaplan, 8/e, p 1033.)* Tardive dyskinesia (TD) is characterized by involuntary choreoathetoid movements of the face, trunk, and extremities. Tardive dyskinesia is associated with prolonged use of medications that block dopamine receptors, most commonly antipsychotic medications. Typical antipsychotic medications (such as perphenazine) and, in particular, high-potency drugs carry the highest risk of TD. Atypical antipsychotics are thought to be less likely to cause this disorder.

208. The answer is b. *(Kaplan, 8/e, p 1033.)* Although tardive dyskinesia (which the man in the question has) often emerges while patients are taking a steady dosage of medication, it is even more likely to emerge when the dosage is reduced. This is called withdrawal dyskinesia, although it is indistinguishable from tardive dyskinesia. Once tardive dyskinesia is recognized, physicians should consider reducing the dosage of the dopamine receptor antagonist or even stopping the medication altogether. While tardive dyskinesia is often considered permanent, some reduction in movements is seen in most patients by 18 months after the discontinuation of antipsychotics.

209. The answer is c. *(Ebert, p 75.)* The risk of developing schizophrenia in first-degree relatives of schizophrenic patients is elevated compared to the risk of the general population (0.9%). Parents of schizophrenic patients have a lifetime prevalence of 5.9%, and siblings have a prevalence of 10%. Children of schizophrenics have a lifetime prevalence of 12.8%.

210. The answer is e. *(Kaplan, 8/e, p 546.)* This patient is presenting with a major depression with psychotic features. For over 2 weeks (the minimum for the diagnosis), the patient has been complaining of anhedonia, crying, anergia, decreased concentration, 25-lb weight loss, and insomnia with early morning awakening. She also has somatic delusions that are mood congruent and an auditory hallucination. The presence of psychotic phenomena that follow a clear mood disorder picture makes the diagnosis of major depression with psychotic features the most likely.

211. The answer is c. *(Kaplan, 8/e, pp 504–508.)* Schizophreniform disorder and chronic schizophrenia differ only in the duration of the symptoms and the fact that the impaired social or occupational functioning associated with chronic schizophrenia is not required to diagnose schizophreniform disorder. As with schizophrenia, schizophreniform disorder is characterized by the presence of delusions, hallucinations, disorganized thoughts and speech, and negative symptoms. The total duration of the illness, including prodromal and residual phases, is at least 1 month and less than 6 months. Approximately one-third of patients diagnosed with schizophreniform disorder experience a full recovery, while the rest progress to schizophrenia and schizoaffective disorder.

Depending on the predominance of particular symptoms, four subtypes of schizophrenia are recognized: paranoid, disorganized, catatonic, and residual. The man in the question presents with the classical symptoms of paranoid schizophrenia. This subtype of schizophrenia is characterized by prominent hallucinations and delusional ideations with a relative preservation of affect and cognitive functions. Delusions are usually grandiose or persecutory or both, organized around a central coherent theme. Hallucinations, usually auditory, are frequent and related to the delusional theme.

Anxiety, anger, argumentativeness, and aloofness are often present. Paranoid schizophrenia tends to develop later in life and it is associated with a better prognosis.

212. The answer is a. *(Kaplan, 8/e, pp 512–520.)* The main feature of delusional disorder is the presence of one or more nonbizarre delusions without deterioration of psychosocial functioning and in the absence of bizarre or odd behavior. Auditory and visual hallucinations, if present, are not prominent and are related to the delusional theme. Tactile and olfactory hallucinations may also be present if they are incorporated in the delusional system (such as feeling insects crawling over the skin in delusions of infestation). Subtypes of delusional disorder include erotomanic, grandiose, jealous, persecutory, and somatic (delusions of being infested with parasites, of emitting a bad odor, of having AIDS). Delusional disorder usually manifests in middle or late adult life and has a fluctuating course with periods of remissions and relapses.

213. The answer is b. *(Kaplan, 8/e, pp 456–491.)* The essential characteristics of the disorganized type of schizophrenia are disorganized speech and behavior, flat or inappropriate affect, great functional impairment, and inability to perform basic activities such as showering or preparing meals. Grimacing along with silly and odd behavior and mannerisms is common. Hallucinations and delusions, if present, are fragmented and not organized in a coherent theme. This subtype is associated with poor premorbid functions, early insidious onset, and a progressive course without remissions.

214. The answer is d. *(Kaplan, 8/e, p 469.)* Catatonic schizophrenia is characterized by marked psychomotor disturbances including prolonged immobility, posturing, extreme negativism (the patient actively resists any attempts made to change his or her position) or waxy flexibility (the patient maintains the position in which he or she is placed), mutism, echolalia (repetition of words said by another person), and echopraxia (repetition of movements made by another person). Periods of immobility and mutism can alternate with periods of extreme agitation (catatonic excitement).

215. The answer is a. *(Kaplan, 8/e, pp 508–509.)* Schizoaffective disorder is diagnosed when the required criteria for schizophrenia are met (delusions, hallucination, disorganized speech or behavior, and/or negative symptoms; duration of the disturbance, including prodromal and residual period, of at least 6 months with at least 1 month of active symptoms) and the patient experiences at some point in the course of the illness a major depressive episode or a manic episode. The man in the question meets all these criteria. Delusional disorder is not accompanied by decline in functions or significant affective symptoms. Individuals with schizoid personality disorder do not experience psychotic symptoms. Bipolar disorder is differentiated from schizoaffective disorder by the absence of periods of psychosis accompanied by prominent affective symptoms.

216. The answer is b. *(Kaplan, 8/e, p 251.)* Formal thought disorder is common in schizophrenia, although it is also encountered in mania and depression. Forms of formal thought disorder characterized by a disturbance of the flow of ideation include thought blocking, poverty of speech, and flight of ideas. Disturbances of thought continuity include circumstantiality, tangentiality, clang association, loose associations, derailment, and echolalia. Concrete and illogical thinking are also forms of formal thought disorder. Although certain forms of formal thought disorder are more frequently associated with specific psychiatric disorders (for example, tangentiality, flight of ideas, and clang association in mania, and illogical thinking and loose association in schizophrenia), no form of thought disorder appears to be disorder specific. Delusions, obsessions, and ideas of reference are disturbances of thought content.

217. The answer is d. *(Kaplan, 8/e, pp 1071–1073.)* Clozapine is an atypical antipsychotic agent that treats both the positive and negative symptoms of schizophrenia while causing a minimum of extrapyramidal adverse effects. The principal drawbacks of clozapine are the need to monitor closely for agranulocytosis (through the use of pretreatment and weekly WBCs) and the relatively high risk of seizure and orthostatic hypotension.

218. The answer is b. *(Kaplan, 8/e, pp 508–509.)* Schizoaffective disorder is diagnosed when the required criteria for schizophrenia are met (delusions, hallucination, disorganized speech or behavior, and/or negative symptoms; duration of the disturbance, including prodromal and residual period, of at least 6 months with at least 1 month of active symptoms) and the patient experiences at some point in the course of the illness a major depressive episode or a manic episode. The woman in the question meets all these criteria. She has continuing psychotic symptomatology, interspersed with episodes of a major mood disorder. Notably, she has never had the mood symptoms without the psychotic symptoms, ruling out major depression with psychosis as the diagnosis. Delusional disorder is not accompanied by decline in functions or significant affective symptoms. Individuals with schizoid personality disorder do not experience psychotic symptoms. Bipolar disorder is differentiated from schizoaffective disorder by the absence of periods of psychosis accompanied by prominent affective symptoms.

219. The answer is a. *(Kaplan, 8/e, pp 512–520.)* This patient is suffering from an erotomanic delusion—the delusion of having a special relationship with another person, often someone famous.

220. The answer is d. *(Kaplan, 8/e, p 1076.)* The schizophrenic patient in the question manifests a prevalence of negative symptoms (flat affect, abulia, lack of motivation). Two antipsychotic medications have been proved to be effective for negative symptoms: clozapine and olanzapine. However, due to clozapine's high risk for agranulocytosis, its use is limited to refractory cases of schizophrenia, severe tardive dyskinesia, and psychotic symptoms in patients with Parkinson's disease.

221. The answer is d. *(Kaplan, 8/e, p 881.)* This patient has experienced a common side effect associated with the use of low-potency neuroleptics, in particular chlorpromazine. These medications have a photosensitization effect and cause sunburn, patchy discoloration of the skin, and rashes when the patients are exposed to the sun without adequate protection (sunscreens, hats, long sleeves).

222. The answer is d. *(Kaplan, 8/e, p 1033.)* Tardive dyskinesia often improves when the dosage of neuroleptic is decreased or stopped. When these interventions are not effective or are not possible due to the severity of the patient's disorder, olanzapine is the treatment of choice. All the other medications listed are typical antipsychotics, which have just as high a risk for TD as haloperidol.

223. The answer is b. *(Ebert, p 273.)* There is strong evidence that without continuous treatment, virtually all schizophrenic patients relapse within 12 to 24 months. Injectable depot medications such as haloperidol decanoate

Schizophrenia and Other Psychotic Disorders **Answers** 143

and fluphenazine decanoate are effective in decreasing the rate of relapse in patients who are not compliant with oral medication.

224. The answer is c. *(Kaplan, 8/e, p 252.)* A delusion is defined as a firmly held false belief that is not shared by other people in the same social and cultural group and is firmly held against evidence that disproves the belief. Delusions are classified as disturbances of thought content and they are found in a wide variety of psychotic conditions other than schizophrenia, including organic disorders, states of intoxication, and mood disorders. Although certain types of delusions are more common in certain disorders (delusions of being controlled by external agents in schizophrenia and grandiose delusions in mania), delusions are not diagnostically specific. Hallucinations are disorders of perception in which a sensory sensation is described when no such stimulus exists.

225. The answer is c. *(Ebert, p 276.)* Suicide is a significant risk factor for schizophrenic patients, and it has been calculated that approximately 9 to 13% of these patients commit suicide due to despair and depression or in response to command hallucinations or persecutory delusions.

226. The answer is d. *(Kaplan, 8/e, pp 520–523.)* Brief psychotic disorder is characterized by the sudden appearance of delusions, hallucinations, and disorganized speech or behavior, usually following a severe stressor. The episode lasts at least 1 day and less than 1 month and is followed by full spontaneous remission. For the woman in the question, the psychotic episode was clearly precipitated by the death of her children. Schizophreniform disorder is differentiated from brief psychotic disorder by temporal factors (in schizophreniform disorder, symptoms are required to last more than 1 month) and lack of association with a stressor. Posttraumatic stress disorder has a more chronic course and is characterized by affective, dissociative, and behavioral symptoms.

227. The answer is e. *(Kaplan, 8/e, pp 500–501.)* Postpartum psychosis is a rare event (1 to 2 per 1000 postpartum women). There is believed to be a close relationship between postpartum psychosis and the mood disorders. Restlessness, disorganized behavior, derealization, hallucinations, and delusions develop rapidly within the first 2 to 4 weeks after delivery. Delusional beliefs and hallucinations often center on the infant. Infanticide is relatively uncommon (4%), but risk for suicide is very high. Psychosocial stressors play an important role in the development of postpartum disorders, and many studies have proved that stressful events during pregnancy increase the risk for postpartum depression and psychosis.

228. The answer is a. *(Ebert, p 266.)* Schizophrenia affects 1% of the adult population. The incidence is comparable in all societies. The 1-year incidence rate is 0.2 per 1000.

229. The answer is d. *(Ebert, p 277.)* Factors predicting a good outcome in schizophrenia include age at onset of 20 to 25, possibly female gender, middle to high socioeconomic status, and a stable occupational record. Other adverse social factors are missing and the family history is one of affective disorder, not schizophrenia. In addition, precipitating factors are usually present, and the onset of the disease is rapid, not insidious, in patients with good outcome schizophrenia.

230. The answer is d. *(Ebert, p 270.)* Amphetamine intoxication can result in a psychosis very closely resembling acute paranoid schizophrenia, with symptoms including paranoid delusions and visual hallucinations. Some investigators feel that prominent visual hallucinations and a relative absence of thought disorder are more characteristic of amphetamine psychosis, but other investigators feel the symptoms are indistinguishable. Other drugs that produce psychoses similar to schizophrenia include phencyclidine (PCP) and lysergic acid diethylamide (LSD).

231. The answer is c. *(Ebert, p 267.)* Gender differences in schizophrenia have been repeatedly demonstrated. The lifetime risk for schizophrenia is the same in males and females, but males tend to have an earlier peak age of onset (18 to 25 years vs. 26 to 45 years for females) and a poorer outcome, because male patients tend to have a poorer response to neuroleptic medication than do female patients.

232. The answer is a. *(Ebert, p 262.)* Frieda Fromm-Reichmann followed the interpersonal school founded by Harry Stack Sullivan and believed that schizophrenia was the outcome of an inadequate mother-child relationship in which the mother was aloof, overly protective, or hostile. She postulated that faulty mothering leads to anxiety and distrust of others, causing people who develop schizophrenia to withdraw from interpersonal exchanges.

This theory has been discredited by recent research that supports the notion that schizophrenia is a brain disorder caused by the convergence of multiple environmental and genetic factors. However, subsequent study of the effect of expressed emotion (family members expressive of hostility and overly controlling) do show that this behavior leads to an increase in relapse rates.

233. The answer is d. *(Kaplan, 8/e, pp 456–491.)* Self-induced water intoxication should always be considered in the differential diagnosis of confusional states and seizures in schizophrenic patients. As many as 20% of patients with a diagnosis of schizophrenia drink excessive amounts of water. At least 4% of these patients suffer from chronic hyponatremia and recurrent acute water intoxication. Medications that cause excessive water retention, such as lithium and carbamazepine, can aggravate the symptomatology.

234–237. The answers are 234-b, 235-a, 236-d, 237-g. *(Ebert, p 289. Kaplan, 8/e, p 499.)* Amok refers to a dissociative episode characterized by violent agitation and aggressive and homicidal behavior. The episode is precipitated by a perceived slight or insult and is preceded by a period of brooding. Amok was first described in Malaysia. Koro is seen in South and East Asia and is characterized by a sudden and intense anxiety connected to the belief that the penis is receding into the body and that death will follow when it has totally disappeared. Nervios is a common disorder in South America and among the Latino population in the United States. Nervios is characterized by a wide range of symptoms of emotional distress, somatic complaints, and decreased ability to function. Headaches, stomach problems, insomnia, irritability, tearfulness, trembling, and vertigo are only some of the symptoms associated with this disorder. Nervios is a very broad syndrome that occurs in individuals with no mental disorder as well as those with a variety of depressive and anxiety disorders. Mal de ojo is a disorder found in Mediterranean populations and is thought by people affected to have been caused by the "evil eye." Symptoms include vomiting, fever, and restless sleep. Sangue dormido, a syndrome described among Portuguese Cape Verdians, includes numbness, tremor, paralysis, convulsions, strokes, and heart attacks. Dhat is characterized by anxiety, hypochondriac concern about semen discharge, and fatigue. It is found in India. Windigo is a rare psychotic state manifested by certain North American Indian tribes in which patients believe that they are possessed by a demon or monster that murders and eats human flesh.

238. The answer is d. *(Ebert, p 288.)* Autoscopic psychosis has as its main symptom the visual hallucination of a transparent phantom of one's own body. Capgras syndrome (delusion of doubles) is a fixed belief that familiar persons have been replaced by identical imposters who behave identically to the original person. Lyncanthropy is the delusion that the person is a werewolf or other animal. Cotard syndrome is the false perception of having lost everything, including money, status, strength, and health, but also internal organs. Folie à deux is a shared psychotic disorder in which one person develops psychotic symptoms similar to the ones a long-term partner has been experiencing.

Psychotherapies

Questions

DIRECTIONS: Each item below contains a question or incomplete statement followed by suggested responses. Select the **one best** response to each question.

Items 239–240

239. A 40-year-old woman with a history of chaotic interpersonal relationships enters psychoanalytic psychotherapy. She alternates between periods in which she idealizes the therapist and the progress of the therapy and periods of unrelenting anger when she is convinced that the therapist is unhelpful and that the therapeutic work is worthless. Which defense mechanism is being used by the patient in this scenario?

a. Reaction formation
b. Denial
c. Projection
d. Projective identification
e. Splitting

240. This defense mechanism is most commonly seen in which of the following diagnoses?

a. Borderline personality disorder
b. Histrionic personality disorder
c. Narcissistic personality disorder
d. Major depression
e. Obsessive-compulsive disorder

241. In psychoanalytic theory, which of the following statements is true of the phenomenon of transference?

a. It only occurs in the therapeutic relationship between patient and therapist
b. When it occurs, it always has a negative effect on the therapy
c. It interferes with the reconstruction of the patient's past
d. It is the result of the displacement of old feelings and beliefs onto another
e. It only manifests itself during patients' dreams

Items 242–243

242. A 25-year-old woman suffering from recurrent major depression becomes very distressed when her supervisor asks her to revise a project she has been working on for weeks. "I don't do anything right. I must be the most incompetent person in the firm. I will lose my job for sure!" she states, sobbing, to her therapist. According to the cognitive model, her depression is a consequence of which of the following problems?
 a. Anger turned toward the self
 b. Early parental empathic failure
 c. Unresolved oedipal complex
 d. Maladaptive negative beliefs
 e. Difficulty mastering the challenges of adulthood

243. In the cognitive model, which of the following interventions should the therapist begin with this patient?
 a. Ask the patient to return to her workplace and take on another project
 b. Tell the patient that she is feeling this way because her self-esteem is low
 c. Tell the patient that she is blowing the episode out of proportion
 d. Ask the patient to talk about her feelings of humiliation and devastation
 e. Ask the patient to write down her thoughts so that the two can discuss them

244. Which of the following statements is true with regard to the development of a transference neurosis in psychoanalytic therapy?
 a. It only occurs in the very early stages of treatment
 b. It only occurs in patients with severe psychopathology
 c. It is an integral part of the therapeutic process
 d. It usually involves the reenactment of adolescent power struggles
 e. It involves negative, but not positive, feelings toward the therapist

245. Why is psychotherapy for personality disorders so difficult to do successfully?
 a. The traits are often ego-dystonic
 b. The patients are usually too sick to use psychotherapy
 c. These disorders respond better to medication than psychotherapy
 d. The patients often see their problems as the result of others, not their own
 e. The patients do not have the ego strength for confrontation or interpretation

246. Under hypnosis, a woman who was sexually abused by her father during most of her childhood sobbingly pleads, "Daddy, please don't hurt me." At the end of the session, she states she understands better why she always had a strong sense of revulsion when any man touched her. This experience is an example of which of the following?
a. Conversion disorder
b. Histrionic personality traits
c. Visual hallucination
d. Reaction formation
e. Abreaction

247. A patient in psychodynamic therapy has been coming late to the last few sessions and complaining in the sessions that he has nothing to talk about. His therapist points out that they were making very rapid progress into uncovering some of the difficult thoughts and feelings the patient had about his parents up until several weeks ago. This recent change in the patient's behavior is an example of what therapeutic principle?
a. Countertransference
b. Ego strength
c. Abreaction
d. Projective identification
e. Resistance

248. A 24-year-old woman with bulimia joins an eating disorder support group at the advice of her psychiatrist. After years of being deeply ashamed of her disorder and keeping it secret, she is relieved to hear that others in the group have binged and purged as she had. Which of the following terms best describes this phenomenon, which is common in self-help groups?
a. Universalization
b. Group cohesion
c. Multiple transference
d. Shared belief system
e. Validation

249. A 22-year-old student is in therapy because he has a long history of chaotic interpersonal relationships, episodes of psychosis, and multiple hospitalizations. He has had three suicide attempts, mostly precipitated by his feeling overwhelmed in some social setting. He comes to his therapist greatly upset and anxious one session because he forgot to study some material that will be on an upcoming exam. The therapist reminds the patient that he has done well on previous exams, and suggests that they spend their time in the session devising a study plan for the time the patient has left before the test. These interventions are commonly used in which of the following therapies?

a. Psychoanalysis
b. Object relation psychotherapy
c. Cognitive-behavioral therapy
d. Supportive psychotherapy
e. Interpersonal psychotherapy

250. In psychoanalytic psychotherapy, which of the following statements best illustrates the concept of countertransference?

a. It is an essential component of the therapy
b. It is harmful to the process when it occurs
c. When it occurs, the therapist should refer the patient to another physician
d. When it occurs, the therapist should enter therapy him- or herself
e. It is an indication that the therapist dislikes the patient

251. Client-centered psychotherapy stresses which of the following characteristics in the therapist?

a. Ability to remain neutral
b. Ability to give unconditional positive regard
c. Ability to confront and set limits
d. Ability to give sound advice
e. Ability to perform hypnosis

252. A 35-year-old physician with a successful private practice is in therapy for long-standing feelings of inadequacy and doubts about her skills. She is eventually able to trace these feelings back to her perfectionistic mother's constant disapproval. She describes in one session feeling intensely ashamed and exposed when a colleague of hers pointed out a minor diagnostic error that she had made. If the therapist is using Kohut's model of therapy, which of the following responses should be made to the patient's distress?
 a. Empathy with the patient
 b. Interpretation of the patient's childhood experiences
 c. Silence to allow the patient to free-associate
 d. Teaching the patient a deep muscle relaxation exercise
 e. Asking the patient to make a list of all the times she had made a correct diagnosis

253. A young man in psychoanalysis has recurrent dreams of snakes shedding their skins. What are these images called by Jungian psychotherapists?
 a. Phallic representations
 b. Archetypes
 c. Illusions
 d. Primary process
 e. Manifest content of a dream

254. Which of the following topics is principally focused on in cognitive therapy?
 a. Unconscious and repressed memories
 b. Faulty ideas and beliefs
 c. Transference manifestations
 d. Dream interpretation
 e. Relaxation techniques

255. A patient perceives his analyst as wise, caring, and helpful. During his session, he talks at length about his warm feelings toward the therapist. Which of the following avenues should the analyst take?
 a. Tell the patient that he does not really feel this way—he is experiencing transference
 b. Tell the patient that his positive feelings cannot be reciprocated
 c. Tell the patient that these feelings are not helpful in the service of the therapy
 d. Tell the patient that underneath the positive feelings are undoubtedly negative ones
 e. Ask the patient to explore related feelings he has about the topic

DIRECTIONS: Each group of questions below consists of lettered options followed by a set of numbered items. For each numbered item, select the **one** lettered option with which it is **most** closely associated. Each lettered option may be used once, more than once, or not at all.

Items 256–262

Match the correct defense mechanism with each patient's actions.

a. Distortion
b. Repression
c. Reaction formation
d. Sublimation
e. Somatization
f. Intellectualization
g. Suppression
h. Isolation of affect
i. Introjection
j. Projection
k. Identification with the aggressor
l. Projective identification
m. Denial
n. Displacement

256. A patient starts complaining of chest pain and coughing whenever her therapist confronts her. She insists, however, that she is not at all distressed or angry. **(CHOOSE 1 DEFENSE MECHANISM)**

257. A woman feels jealous and hurt when, at a family gathering, her husband flirts with her younger cousin. She makes a conscious decision to put her feelings aside and to wait for a more appropriate moment to confront her husband and convey her emotions. **(CHOOSE 1 DEFENSE MECHANISM)**

258. A young man gets into an argument with his teacher. Although very upset, he remains silent as she chastises him severely and calls him a failure as a student. Once he gets home from school, the young man picks a fight with his younger brother over nothing and begins screaming at him. **(CHOOSE 1 DEFENSE MECHANISM)**

Psychotherapies 153

259. A 34-year-old man is deeply envious of his younger but much more successful brother. Although it is difficult for him to admit, he believes the younger brother was their parents' favorite as well. He tells his friends that his younger brother is envious of his good looks and successes with women, even though there is some evidence to the fact that this is not so. **(CHOOSE 1 DEFENSE MECHANISM)**

260. A 28-year-old woman is in psychotherapy for a long-standing depressed mood and poor self-esteem. One day during the session, the therapist yawns because she is very tired, though she is interested in what the patient has to say. The patient immediately bursts into tears, saying that the therapist must be bored and uninterested in her and must have been for quite some time. **(CHOOSE 1 DEFENSE MECHANISM)**

261. A man who was beaten as a child by his parents for every small infraction nonetheless idealizes them and describes them as "good parents who did not spoil their children." He is baffled and angry when he is ordered to start parenting classes after the school nurse reports that his children consistently come to school with bruises. **(CHOOSE 1 DEFENSE MECHANISM)**

262. A 52-year-old man is hospitalized after a severe myocardial infarction. On the second day in the hospital, when his physician comes by on rounds, the patient insists on jumping out of bed and doing several push-ups to show the physician that "they can't keep a good man down—there is nothing wrong with me!" **(CHOOSE 1 DEFENSE MECHANISM)**

Items 263–265

263. A 7-year-old autistic mentally retarded boy is brought to the psychologist because the staff of the residential center in which the boy lives are concerned about the severity of his self-destructive behavior. Which of the following pieces of information would a psychologist conducting a functional behavioral analysis be most interested in?
a. The staff's feelings toward the boy
b. The parents' psychiatric history
c. The boy's IQ
d. The consequences to the boy of his behavior
e. The quality of the boy's early interactions with his mother

264. The psychologist evaluating the boy observes him at his day school. She notes that this behavior dramatically increases when his teachers are involved with other students, and it causes them to turn their behavior away from the other students and toward the boy, either to scold him or restrain him. In a behavioral model, which of the following is the best descriptor of the teachers' responses?

a. Aversive stimulus
b. Reinforcer
c. Conditioned stimulus
d. Secondary gain
e. Reminder

265. The psychologist recommends to the teachers that they ignore the boy's self-injurious behavior. After 3 weeks, the target behaviors are greatly decreased. Which of the following mechanisms is involved in this behavioral improvement?

a. Counterconditioning
b. Suppression
c. Habituation
d. Desensitization
e. Extinction

266. A 34-year-old woman comes to a psychiatrist because she has an extreme fear of heights. After being taught relaxation techniques, she is accompanied up a staircase and is asked to look down from her position at increasingly higher spots while performing her relaxation exercises. Which of the following is the technique that is being employed?

a. Desensitization
b. Reframing
c. Contingency management
d. Flooding
e. Operant conditioning

267. A 38-year-old man comes to see a psychiatrist because of conflicts with his new wife and the resulting anxiety and depression that this has caused him. On evaluation, he is found to have a paranoid delusion. Therapy is suggested as part of the recommended treatment. Which of the following therapies is likely to be contraindicated?
a. Family therapy
b. Supportive psychotherapy
c. Hypnosis
d. Cognitive therapy
e. Progressive muscle relaxation

268. A patient in psychotherapy is always anxious to please. Recently, he has stated that he has begun to feel frightened in the presence of the therapist and that he has had fantasies about the analyst attacking him. Subsequently, the patient talks about his father and of his lifelong struggle to please him at any cost. After listening to these comments, the therapist says that the patient's fantasies about him appear to be closely connected with the patient's way of relating to his father. The therapist also says that the passive and compliant relationship the patient has with his idealized father may represent a reaction to his fear of his father's retaliation. These comments represent which kind of therapeutic intervention?
a. Confrontation
b. Interpretation
c. Clarification
d. Desensitization
e. Flooding

269. Which of the following characteristics is primarily related to a patient's hypnotizability?
a. Patient compliance
b. Patient suggestibility
c. Patient ego strength
d. Therapist's power of persuasion
e. Therapist countertransference

270. The parents of a 20-year-old schizophrenic are having difficulty dealing with their son's decline in function. Once a good student with friends and a social life, the son now spends his days barricaded in his room, mumbling to himself or watching the street with binoculars. Which of the following family interventions would be most helpful in this situation?

a. Teaching the parents about reducing expressed emotions in the family's interactions
b. Unmasking the family game and freeing the identified patient from the role of symptom bearer
c. Encouraging the parents to openly discuss their feelings of loss and disappointment with their son
d. Discussing the secondary gains provided by the son's symptoms
e. Discussing the parents' marital problems and how the son's disorder affects them

271. A 27-year-old man comes to the physician with the chief complaint of premature ejaculation. He has been married for 4 months but has been unable to consummate the marriage due to his sexual problem. Which of the following treatments will be most helpful for the man's premature ejaculation?

a. Exploration of the husband's relationship with his domineering mother
b. Discussion of the wife's unexpressed masochistic fantasies
c. Interpretation of the husband's dreams
d. Squeeze technique and stop-and-start technique
e. Instructing the husband to masturbate several times a day with the goal to reach an orgasm as fast as possible

272. A 49-year-old man comes to the doctor with high blood pressure and anxiety. Preferring to try something other than medication at first, the patient agrees to try another approach. He is attached to an apparatus that measures skin temperature and emits a tone proportional to the temperature. Which of the following techniques is being used with this patient?

a. Hypnosis
b. Progressive muscle relaxation
c. Autogenic techniques
d. Placebo
e. Biofeedback

273. A 16-year-old boy is hospitalized on the adolescent ward of a psychiatric unit for new-onset psychotic behavior. The boy consistently avoids bathing and taking care of his personal hygiene, and is resistant to changing this behavior. He is put on a system by which he earns points for accomplishing various aspects of personal hygiene. These points can be redeemed at the snack shop, or they can purchase extra activity passes. Which of the following treatment techniques is being used with this patient?
a. Token economy
b. Social skills training
c. Classical conditioning
d. Reward system
e. Cognitive remediation

274. A high school teacher is respected and loved by both his students and his colleagues because he can easily defuse tense moments with an appropriate light remark and he always seems to be able to find something funny in any situation. Which of the following defense mechanisms is this man using?
a. Displacement
b. Denial
c. Reaction formation
d. Humor
e. Suppression

Items 275–278

For each patient, select the one most appropriate therapeutic option.
a. Psychoanalysis
b. Brief individual psychotherapy
c. Cognitive therapy
d. Behavioral therapy
e. Family therapy
f. Group therapy

275. A young woman with no previous psychiatric history develops an incapacitating fear of driving after being involved in a minor automobile accident. **(CHOOSE 1 THERAPEUTIC OPTION)**

276. A 40-year-old, married, successful businessman with a satisfying family life becomes preoccupied with thoughts of becoming involved with a younger woman. He has no prior psychiatric history and no other complaints. **(CHOOSE 1 THERAPEUTIC OPTION)**

277. A 16-year-old girl begins acting out sexually and skipping school. These symptoms coincide with the onset of frequent arguments between her parents, who have been threatening marital separation. **(CHOOSE 1 THERAPEUTIC OPTION)**

278. An intelligent 25-year-old single woman who has a successful career complains of multiple failed relationships with men, unhappiness, and a wish to sort out her life. A previous experience in individual psychotherapy was somewhat helpful. **(CHOOSE 1 THERAPEUTIC OPTION)**

279. Which of the following statements best describes the cognitive approach to the treatment of panic disorder?
a. Taking the patient to a crowded place and preventing escape until the patient's anxiety has peaked
b. Teaching the patient to hyperventilate as soon as he or she starts feeling anxious
c. Educating the patient about the harmless nature of the physical symptoms experienced during a panic attack
d. Taking the patient through a series of imaginary exposures in the therapist's office
e. Replying empathically to the patient about the suffering that must be endured with panic attacks

280. A physician with a very busy practice feels satisfied and fulfilled when he can make a difference in the lives of his patients. Which of the following defense mechanisms is being used, according to psychoanalytic theory?
a. Reaction formation
b. Altruism
c. Sublimation
d. Asceticism
e. Idealization

281. An 18-year-old girl comes to the psychiatrist with the chief complaint of pulling out her hair in patches when she is anxious or upset. She is taught to make a tight fist whenever she has this impulse rather than pull out her hair. Which of the following techniques is this?
a. Habit reversal training
b. Extinction
c. Simple conditioning
d. Flooding
e. Desensitization

282. A 34-year-old man comes to the psychiatrist with the chief complaint of marital problems, which seemed to begin just after the death of his mother. In therapy, it is discovered that the patient had an intensively ambivalent relationship with his mother. However, when he discusses his mother, the patient appears unemotional and detached. Which of the following defense mechanisms is this patient using?
a. Projection
b. Isolation of affect
c. Splitting
d. Reaction formation
e. Projective identification

283. Freud wrote about the concept of abstinence in his guidelines for psychoanalytic psychotherapy. Which of the following best describes this concept?
a. A prohibition on sexual relationships with patients
b. A recommendation on professional behavior for analysts
c. A prohibition against therapists getting their needs met at the expense of the patient
d. The requirement that therapists function as a "blank screen" during sessions
e. A requirement of the therapist to frustrate the patient's regressive wishes

284. Interpersonal psychotherapy was developed in the 1970s by Gerard Klerman as a time-limited treatment for major depressive disorders. Which of the following does this type of therapy focus on?
a. Childhood losses
b. Current relationships
c. Intrapsychic conflicts
d. Making the unconscious conscious
e. Correcting distorted beliefs

285. A young woman with obsessive-compulsive disorder has suffered from contamination fears for years, and now her hands are raw from so much washing. Her therapist takes her to the bathroom and asks her to touch the toilet seat. Afterward, he stops her from washing her hands. The patient's anxiety rapidly increases, and after a peak, declines. Which of the following is the name of this technique?

a. Exposure
b. Desensitization
c. Counterconditioning
d. Operational conditioning
e. Functional behavioral analysis

Psychotherapies

Answers

239–240. The answers are 239-e, 240-a. *(Ebert, p 46.)* The concept of splitting as an unconscious ego defense was first introduced by Melanie Klein and later elaborated by Otto Kernberg, two of the main theorists of the object relation movement. Although this defense is occasionally used by patients with neurotic disturbances, splitting is mostly encountered in more severely disturbed patients, such as patients with personality disorders and, in particular, borderline personality disorder. According to the object relation theory, patients with severe personality disorders due to faulty parenting during infancy have not been able to form stable and realistic intrapsychic representations of themselves and of the important people in their lives. Instead of seeing themselves and others as consistent entities containing both good and bad traits, they perceive the negative and positive aspects as separate, irreconcilable parts. Splitting, by allowing the manifestation of only one side of the ambivalence at a time, preserves the good objects, which otherwise, in the patient's experience, would consistently risk being contaminated and neutralized by the bad objects. In the case described, in order to preserve her view of her therapist as helpful and kind (and her positive feelings toward him), the patient has to split the less than perfect traits of the therapist as well as all her negative thoughts and feelings toward him. Unfortunately, when disappointments, real or imagined, bring the negative side of the ambivalence into focus, patients who use splitting as a main defense temporarily lose contact with the positive side.

241. The answer is d. *(Ebert, p 44.)* Transference, according to the classical Freudian psychoanalytic theory, refers to the projection of feelings, thoughts, and attitudes once connected to important figures in the patient's past onto the analyst. Due to transference, patients unconsciously reenact with the analyst old scripts instead of consciously remembering and processing the past. Freud did not distinguish between the real patient-analyst relationship and transference, and he did not talk about the real traits in the analyst that can affect the transference. In the contemporary psychoanalytic movement, transference is considered a mixture of reality and reenactment, and it is well accepted that the analyst's personal characteristics influence both the quality and the intensity of the transference. Transference is not limited to the patient-analyst relationship but can take place in any meaningful relationship. Transference does not hinder the treatment; on the contrary, the analysis of the transference helps patients understand how their past still affects their emotional reactions and behaviors. Verbal and nonverbal communication, overt behavioral patterns, omissions, and dreams are some of the ways transference manifests itself.

242–243. The answers are 242-d, 243-e. *(Ebert, p 292.)* Cognitive therapy is based on the principle that psychopathology derives from the patient's faulty, distorted beliefs about him- or herself and the world (schemas). Negative schemas derive from past negative experiences and evoke powerful emotions. The goal of cognitive therapy is to replace negative and maladaptive beliefs and thought patterns with more adaptive, positive ones. In this process, called cognitive restructuring, while the patient reviews with the therapist the automatic thoughts that accompany his or her distressing emotions ("Everybody hates me" or "I will never amount to anything"), logical errors are identified, the validity of the negative assumptions is challenged by more realistic evidence ("I have several friends who care for me, so it is not true that everybody hates me"), and alternative explanations for events are explored ("My friend did not ignore me because I am worthless, but, most likely, he was distracted.").

244. The answer is c. *(Kaplan, 8/e, p 887.)* In psychoanalytic theory, transference neurosis refers to the replication of the patient's childhood conflicts and dynamics with the analyst. Transference neurosis takes place in the middle part of therapy and is characterized, on the side of the patient, by intense transferential feelings toward the analyst and regression. The development of transference neurosis is an essential part of the psychoanalytic treatment, because once old conflicts are brought into the present, they can be analyzed, understood, and, finally, resolved.

245. The answer is d. *(Kaplan, 8/e, p 775.)* Although personality disorders cause considerable suffering for patients and people with whom they relate, these patients usually are oblivious to the fact that their characterological traits and maladaptive behaviors create and perpetuate their suffering (e.g., their traits are ego-syntonic). On the contrary, these patients tend to blame others for their difficulties and deny that they have any problems.

Relatives, friends, and co-workers usually have a much better understanding of the patient's dysfunctional traits than the patient has.

246. The answer is e. *(Kaplan, 8/e, p 280.)* Hypnosis is a useful instrument in the treatment of traumatized patients, especially when the memory of the traumatic event or events has been repressed. Through abreaction (or reenactment), the traumatic experience is once again available to the conscious mind, becomes less powerful, and can be gradually integrated into the patient's current view of him- or herself in a meaningful way.

247. The answer is e. *(Kaplan, 8/e, p 888.)* Freud noticed that patients, in spite of their suffering and their overt desire to change, tended to cling to their symptoms and resisted the analyst's efforts to produce insight. He called these powerful internal forces that oppose change resistance. Resistance takes place at any point in the treatment, and particularly when unacceptable impulses or thoughts threaten to come into consciousness or a maladaptive defense mechanism is challenged. Resistance can manifest itself in many different ways, including withholding important thoughts from the analyst, falling silent during sessions, forgetting appointments, forgetting to pay the analyst, falling asleep during session, and considering dropping out of treatment. The possible manifestations of resistance are countless and depend on the patient's defense mechanisms and personality. In other words, the patient's intrapsychic defenses manifest as resistance in the context of his or her interpersonal relationship with the analyst. Freud thought that resistance should be uncovered by the analyst but not challenged or interpreted. Modern analysts believe that resistance should be analyzed through the patient's free associations, supported by the analyst's observations.

248. The answer is a. *(Kaplan, 8/e, p 900.)* Universalization, the awareness that the patient is not alone or unique in his or her suffering and that others share similar symptoms and difficulties, is a powerful healing factor in group therapy. The other items listed are also factors that facilitate the therapeutic group process. Group cohesion refers to the sense that the group is working together toward a common goal. Validation refers to the confirmation of the patient's reality through comparison with other group members' experiences and conceptualizations. Shared belief system refers to the notion that the group may come to have a framework of beliefs and ideas about issues that is common to everyone in the group. Multiple transference refers to the projections of feelings, thoughts, and wishes that belong to the patients' past experiences onto other group members and the group leaders.

249. The answer is d. *(Kaplan, 8/e, p 489.)* Supportive psychotherapy is characterized by an emphasis on the nurturing, caring role of the therapist and a focus on current reality. Although insight-oriented strategies such as interpretations can be used, they are not the main therapeutic instruments. Supportive psychotherapy aims to foster and maintain a positive transference all the time in order to provide the patient with a consistently safe and secure atmosphere. Consolation, advice, reality testing, environmental manipulation, reassurance, and encouragement are strategies commonly used in supportive psychotherapy.

250. The answer is a. *(Kaplan, 8/e, p 888.)* Countertransference, defined as the therapist's transferential response toward the patient, is an important component of the patient-therapist relationship and is practically inevitable during the course of the treatment. Although countertransference can interfere with the treatment occasionally, especially when it is not consciously recognized by the therapist and is acted out, this process is most of the time a useful tool in psychoanalysis. Through a thoughtful analysis of his or her countertransference, the therapist can often obtain useful information about and insight into the patient's experience.

251. The answer is b. *(Kaplan, 8/e, p 231.)* Client-centered psychotherapy was first proposed by Carl Rogers in the 1940s and subsequently gained great popularity. Client-centered therapy is based on the concept that each person has an innate instinct to grow, integrate, and become more functional, as well as an innate capacity to resolve his or her psychological problems, if provided with a facilitative environment. The aim of the therapy is to create a supportive and accepting interpersonal environment that makes the patient feel relaxed, understood, and ready for personal growth. Rogers postulated that three conditions are necessary for the creation of a facilitative relationship: genuineness (the therapist's ability to be real in the relationship with the patient), unconditional positive regard for the patient, and empathic understanding of the patient's experiences.

252. The answer is a. (*Kaplan, 8/e, p 228.*) Heinz Kohut, one of the founders of the Self-Psychology school of psychoanalysis, believed that patients' symptoms stemmed from a fragmented and unstable sense of self caused by unempathic, harsh, or neglectful parenting during the first years of life. According to Kohut, the goal of the therapist is to understand the patient's needs for validation and empathy and meet these needs, at least partially, in the treatment. In contrast, classical psychoanalysis stresses the importance of frustrating the patient's infantile needs, which, in the end, will be renounced and not fulfilled. Although Kohut did not reject the use of the classical tools of psychoanalysis, such as interpretations and free associations, providing a corrective emotional response to the patient was central to his theory.

253. The answer is b. (*Kaplan, 8/e, p 227.*) According to Carl Jung, archetypes are powerful symbolic images that emerge from the collective unconscious, that part of the psychic apparatus that preserves the collective knowledge and experience of humankind. Archetypes emerge in dreams, fantasy, art, and free associations, and their interpretation provides useful insights into the patient's intrapsychic processes. In the scenario described in the question, the snakes shedding their skins are usually interpreted as a symbol for change and renewal. Primary processes, manifest content of dreams, and phallic representations are concepts encountered in Freudian psychoanalytic theories.

254. The answer is b. (*Kaplan, 8/e, pp 919–923.*) Cognitive therapy is based on the concept that psychopathology is a consequence of distorted beliefs and faulty assumptions. Common thinking errors described in the cognitive model are arbitrary inference (drawing a conclusion in the absence of supporting evidence), selective abstraction (focusing on only one small part of a situation or event while ignoring other, usually more positive, aspects), overgeneralization (drawing a general conclusion on the basis of a single incident), magnification (of problems) and minimization (of positive factors), personalization (tendency to relate external events to oneself without reason for doing so), and dichotomous thinking (extreme, black-or-white thinking). Psychoanalysis depends on dream interpretation, transference manifestation, and recovery of repressed memories. Relaxation techniques belong to the realm of behavioral therapy.

255. The answer is e. *(Kaplan, 8/e, p 888.)* Freud felt that unobjectionable positive transference, defined as the patient's perception of the therapist as caring and helpful, is always helpful to the therapeutic process and should not be analyzed. Critics of Freud's theories pointed out that sometimes an overt positive transference may conceal less flattering feelings. Furthermore, patients' positive perceptions of the therapist are not necessarily all projections from past experiences, since the therapist's personality and behavior have powerful effects on the form and content of the transference.

256–262. The answers are 256-e, 257-g, 258-n, 259-j, 260-a, 261-k, 262-m. *(Kaplan, 8/e, pp 220–221.)* In distortion, the external reality is grossly rearranged to conform to internal needs. Repression is the expelling or withholding of an idea or feeling from consciousness. This defense differs from suppression by effecting conscious inhibition of impulses to the point of losing and not just postponing goals. Reaction formation refers to the substitution of an unacceptable feeling or thought with its opposite. Sublimation is the achieving of impulse gratification and the retention of goals by altering a socially objectionable aim or object to a socially acceptable one. Sublimation allows instincts to be channeled rather than blocked or diverted. Sublimation is a mature defense, together with humor, altruism, asceticism, anticipation, and suppression. Somatization is the conversion of psychic derivatives into bodily symptoms and reacting with somatic manifestations rather than psychic ones. Intellectualization is the excessive use of intellectual processes to avoid affective expression or experience. Isolation of affect is the splitting or separation of an idea from the affect that accompanies it but that is repressed. Introjection is the internalization of the qualities of an object. When used as a defense, it can obliterate the distinction between the subject and the object. Projection is the perception of and reaction to unacceptable inner impulses and their derivatives as though they were outside the self. Identification with the aggressor is the adoption of characteristics or behavior of the victim's aggressor as one's own. For example, it is not uncommon for the victim of child abuse to grow up to be an abusive parent him- or herself. Projective identification occurs mostly in borderline personality disorder and consists of three steps: (1) an aspect of the self is projected onto someone else; (2) the projector tries to coerce the other person to identify with what has been projected; (3) the recipient of the projection and the projector feel a sense of oneness or union. Denial is the avoidance of awareness of some painful aspect of reality by negating sensory data. Displacement refers to the shifting of an emotion or a drive from one object to another (for example, the shifting of unacceptable aggressive feelings toward one's parents to the family cat).

263–265. The answers are 263-d, 264-b, 265-e. *(Kaplan, 8/e, pp 149, 151.)* Behavioral analysis is based on the concept that behavior is shaped by its consequences. Behaviors that are followed by desired consequences (positive reinforcers) or that cause the elimination of unpleasant consequences (negative reinforcers) increase the probability that the behavior will happen again. Events that may be reinforcing for some people may be aversive for others. For example, scolding and other types of negative attention can be reinforcing for some individuals and can function as deterrents for others. Behavioral analysis is commonly used to design appropriate behavioral interventions for self-injurious behavior in patients with mental retardation. Observing and quantifying the patient's behavior under various controlled circumstances allows the identification of what reinforces the unwanted behavior in a particular situation. Once the reinforcer is identified, its removal from the environment will cause a decrease or disappearance of the target behavior, a process called extinction. Extinction occurs when the conditioned stimulus is constantly repeated without the unconditioned stimulus until the response evoked by the conditioned stimulus gradually weakens and eventually disappears. In this example, the boy's self-injurious behavior (the conditioned stimulus) will disappear if the unconditioned stimulus (the attention from the teachers) is withdrawn. An aversive stimulus or punishment is any stimulus that, when presented contingently with a behavior, causes the decrease of that behavior. Time-out is a form of aversive stimulus. An unconditioned stimulus—a term derived from the theory of classical conditioning—refers to the stimulus that naturally elicits a certain response (e.g., salivation at the sight of food). The conditioned stimulus is the neutral stimulus that, after being closely associated to an unconditioned stimulus for some time, elicits the same response as the unconditioned stimulus or conditioned response (e.g., nausea elicited by the mere sight of the room where a patient has received chemotherapy in the past).

266. The answer is a. *(Kaplan, 8/e, p 152.)* All behavioral treatments for phobias have in common exposure to the feared stimulus. Desensitization is based on the concept that when the feared stimulus is presented paired with a behavior that induces a state incompatible with anxiety (e.g., deep muscle relaxation), the phobic stimulus loses its power to create anxiety (counterconditioning). This pairing of feared stimulus with a state incompatible with anxiety is called reciprocal inhibition. For desensitization to work, the anxiety elicited by the exposure has to be low. Treatment starts with exposure to stimuli that produce minimal anxiety and proceeds to stimuli with a higher anxiety potential. Operant conditioning refers to the concept that behavior can be modified by changing the antecedents or the consequences of the behavior (contingency management). Flooding is another exposure-based treatment for phobia, based on extinction rather than counterconditioning. Reframing is an intervention used in family therapy and refers to giving a more acceptable meaning to a problematic behavior or situation.

267. The answer is c. (*Kaplan, 8/e, p 918.*) Hypnosis is not recommended for suspicious and paranoid patients, who are likely to respond negatively to the loss of control that hypnosis evokes. These patients usually refuse to cooperate with the hypnotic inductions. Another category of patients who may have unplanned and potentially negative reactions to hypnosis are individuals with a history of trauma, who may undergo spontaneous abreactions.

268. The answer is b. (*Kaplan, 8/e, p 887–888.*) Interpretations, the cornerstone of psychoanalytic psychotherapy, are explanatory statements made by the analyst that link a symptom, a behavior, or a feeling to its unconscious meaning. Ideally, interpretations help the patient become more aware of unconscious material that has come close to the surface. Confrontation and clarification are also used in psychoanalytic psychotherapy. In confrontation, the analyst points out to the patient something that the patient is trying to avoid. Clarification refers to putting together the information the patient has provided so far and reflecting it back to him or her in a more organized and succinct form. Flooding and desensitization are exposure techniques used in behavioral therapy.

269. The answer is b. (*Kaplan, 8/e, p 918.*) The ability to experience trance is connected to the convergence of three factors: absorption, dissociation, and suggestibility. Absorption refers to the ability to focus attention on a detail while reducing peripheral awareness. Dissociation refers to a functional separation of some of the elements of the identity from consciousness. The more the individual's attention is focused on a particular object, the more likely it is that peripheral information will slip out of consciousness. Suggestibility refers to a tendency to accept suggestions or signals with a relative suspension of judgment. High levels of hypnotizability are not connected with psychopathology or character weakness. On the contrary, people with severe psychiatric disturbances often are not hypnotizable.

270. The answer is a. *(Kaplan, 8/e, pp 488–489.)* Family interventions that have been shown to be effective in the treatment of schizophrenic patients include teaching the family members about schizophrenia, emphasizing the importance of keeping the interpersonal communications at a low emotional quotient (schizophrenic patients tend to relapse when exposed to the intense negative emotions of family members), and helping the family learn more adaptive ways to cope with stress. Discussing marital problems in front of the patient and sharing with the patient the distressing details of the parents' own struggles with his or her mental illness are bound to have negative effects. Uncovering the family game was one of the goals of systemic family therapy created by Selvini-Palazzoli and the Milan group. This model was accepted in the 1960s, when schizophrenia was considered the consequence of pathological parenting. In view of what is now known about schizophrenia's biological etiology, this theory is no longer considered valid.

271. The answer is d. *(Kaplan, 8/e, p 697.)* Treatment of sexual dysfunctions relies on specific exercises, called sensate focus exercises, aimed at decreasing anxiety, to teach the couple to give and take pleasure without the pressure of performance and to increase communication between partners. Furthermore, specific problems are addressed with special techniques. The squeeze technique, used to treat premature ejaculation, aims to raise the threshold of penile excitability by firmly squeezing the coronal ridge of the penis, so as to abruptly decrease the level of excitation, at the earliest sensation of impending orgasm. In the start-and-stop technique, stimulation is repeatedly stopped for a few seconds as soon as orgasm is impending and resumed when the level of excitability decreases.

272. The answer is e. *(Kaplan, 8/e, pp 910–911.)* Biofeedback refers to a therapeutic process in which information about the individual's physiological functions, such as blood pressure and heart rate, are monitored electronically and fed back to the individual by means of lights, sounds, or electronic gauges. Biofeedback allows individuals to control a variety of body responses and in turn to modulate pain and the physiological component of unpleasant emotions such as anxiety.

273. The answer is a. *(Ebert, p 529.)* In the token economy model, the desired behavior is reinforced by tokens that can be exchanged for privileges or desired items. In the token economy, as in other interventions aimed at changing behaviors through contingency management, the techniques are implemented by someone other than the patient and require a precise control of the patient's sources of reinforcement. For these reasons, a token economy is usually used for children, at home or in classroom settings, and for retarded or otherwise poorly functioning hospitalized patients.

274. The answer is d. *(Kaplan, p 221.)* Individuals who use humor as a defense mechanism are able to make use of comedy to express feelings and thoughts with potentially disturbing content without experiencing subjective discomfort and without producing an unpleasant effect on others. Humor is a mature defense. Suppression is consciously or semiconsciously postponing attention to a conscious impulse or conflict. In suppression, discomfort is acknowledged but minimized.

275–278. The answers are 275-d, 276-b, 277-e, 278-a. *(Kaplan, 8/e, pp 888–889, 893–894, 904–909, 911–916.)* Behavioral therapy focuses on decreasing or ameliorating people's maladaptive behavior without theorizing about their inner conflicts. Behaviorists look for observable factors that have been learned or conditioned and can therefore be unlearned. In this example, the young woman has developed a phobia of driving after being in an automobile accident. The behavioral therapy indicated here would be teaching the young woman relaxation exercises, then progressively desensitizing her to driving (the stimulus). Brief individual insight-oriented psychotherapy is characterized by a limited, predetermined number of sessions and the fact that the focus of the treatment remains on specific problematic areas in the life of the patient. Deep restructuring of the patient's psychological apparatus is not the goal of brief therapy. Highly motivated patients who function relatively well are good candidates for this type of therapy. Family therapy aims to improve the level of functioning of the family and the individual by altering the interactions among the family members. There are many different approaches to family therapy (psychodynamic, solution-oriented, narrative, systemic, strategic, structural, and transgenerational, to name only a few). Each school focuses on a particular aspect of the family dynamics and uses different techniques to obtain the desired results. For example, the structural school focuses on patterns of engagement-enmeshment and on family boundaries and hierarchies. The solution-oriented approach focuses on solutions and minimizes the importance of problems. Psychoanalytic psychotherapy is suited to patients with relatively good ego strengths, normal or superior intelligence, ability to abstract and think symbolically, and a genuine wish to understand themselves. Although Freud had originally restricted the indications for psychoanalysis to patients with neuroses of a hysterical, phobic, or obsessive-compulsive nature, it is now felt that this type of therapy benefits a much larger range of patients, including patients with depressive and anxiety disorders, high-functioning borderline and narcissistic personality disorders, avoidant personality disorder, and obsessive-compulsive personality disorder. Psychoanalysis is also helpful for individuals who do not have a psychiatric diagnosis but experience problems with intimacy, interpersonal relationships, assertiveness, self-esteem, and so forth.

279. The answer is c. *(Kaplan, 8/e, pp 919–920.)* The cognitive treatment of panic disorder focuses on the patient's tendency to make catastrophic interpretations about body sensations or states of mind. This approach includes a careful exploration of the patient's bodily symptoms before and during the panic attack and of the automatic thoughts that accompany them, in addition to an educational component with regard to the fact that, although terrifying, panic attack symptoms are not fatal. Other more realistic interpretations of symptoms are discussed, and the patient is encouraged to come up with less catastrophic scenarios ("Even if I have a panic attack in a store, the world does not end."). Exposure techniques are part of behavioral therapy. Empathy with the patient's suffering is a necessary element of all doctor-patient interactions, but in this case it does not represent a specific therapeutic technique.

280. The answer is b. *(Kaplan, 8/e, p 220.)* Altruism, a mature ego defense mechanism, is described as the use of constructive service to others in order to vicariously gratify one's own needs. It may include a form of benign and constructive reaction formation. Sublimation (the achieving of impulse gratification by altering the originally objectionable goal with a more acceptable one) and asceticism (obtaining gratification from renunciation of "base" pleasures) are also mature ego defenses. Reaction formation, described as the transformation of an unconscious, objectionable thought or impulse into its opposite, is a neurotic defense. Idealization refers to perception of others or oneself as totally good at the expense of a more realistic, ambivalent representation. Extremes of idealization and devaluation characterize the defense mechanism known as splitting.

281. The answer is a. *(Kaplan, 8/e, pp 911–916.)* Habit reversal training is used to eliminate dysfunctional habits such as nail biting, tics, and hair pulling. The patient is taught to recognize the triggering stimuli and the behaviors present at the very beginning of the dysfunctional habit (for example, touching the face for hair pulling). Patients are then instructed to perform an action incompatible with the habit whenever they become aware that they are on the verge of pulling their hair or biting their nails. Fist clenching is used as a competitive maneuver in both nail biting and hair pulling. Afterward, the patient is encouraged to engage in a reparatory behavior (brushing the hair or filing the nails) to remove the stimulus that may trigger future events.

282. The answer is b. *(Kaplan, 8/e, p 220.)* Isolation of affect, a neurotic defense, refers to the splitting off of the affective component (usually unpleasant or unacceptable) from an idea or thought. Projection is a primitive, narcissistic defense characterized by the transposition of unacceptable feelings and ideas onto others. In projective identification, after projecting his or her own feelings and impulses onto another person, the individual acts in such a way that the other person feels compelled to act out such feelings (e.g., a patient avoids becoming conscious of his anger by projecting it onto another person, then acts in a way that triggers the other person's angry feelings).

283. The answer is e. *(Kaplan, 8/e, pp 887–889.)* Abstinence refers to Freud's recommendations that transferential wishes should not be satisfied but analyzed. Other technical guidelines Freud provided were neutrality, which refers to the therapist's maintaining a nonjudgmental stance toward the patient, and anonymity, which refers to the therapist's functioning as a mirror or a blank wall where the patient can project his or her fantasies.

284. The answer is b. *(Kaplan, 8/e, p 895.)* Interpersonal therapy is based on the theories of the interpersonal school of Harry Stack Sullivan and Bowlby's research on infantile attachment. Interpersonal therapy in centered on the concept that interpersonal attachments are essential for survival and emotional well-being and that loss of interpersonal relationships causes depression. Interpersonal therapy postulates four interpersonal problem areas: complicated mourning, interpersonal role disputes (conflicts with a significant other), role transition (any change in life status that can cause distress), and interpersonal deficits (lack of social skills). After an initial diagnostic evaluation and a detailed exploration of the patient's current relationship and social functioning, the therapist links the depressive symptoms with the patient's interpersonal situation in the framework of one of the four interpersonal problem areas. The therapy process then focuses on current problems and on what goes on in the patient's life outside the office. The therapist maintains an active, nonneutral, and supportive stance. Role playing and direct advice are often used.

285. The answer is a. *(Ebert, pp 20–21.)* Since compulsive behaviors rapidly neutralize the anxiety created by obsessional thoughts, in the treatment of OCD, response prevention needs to be coupled with exposure to the feared stimulus for the exposure to be effective. Anxiety rapidly rises when the patient is prevented from performing the neutralizing compulsive behavior (e.g., washing hands after touching a contaminated object), but subsequently it declines (extinction). Extinction refers to the progressive disappearance of a behavior or a symptom (in this case, anxiety) when the expected consequence does not happen (getting sick due to contamination). Note the difference between extinction and desensitization: in extinction the anxiety-provoking stimulus is not linked to a calming activity, as occurs in desensitization.

Mood Disorders

Questions

DIRECTIONS: Each item below contains a question or incomplete statement followed by suggested responses. Select the **one best** response to each question.

286. A 32-year-old woman is diagnosed with major depression. What is the chance that her identical twin sister will develop the same disease?
a. 5%
b. 20%
c. 50%
d. 70%
e. 90%

287. A 55-year-old man comes to the psychiatrist with the chief complaint of depressed mood, crying spells, decreased energy, and loss of appetite. One month later he is diagnosed with cancer. Which of the following carcinomas is most likely to manifest with this type of psychiatric symptomatology?
a. Prostatic
b. Renal
c. Gastric
d. Pancreatic
e. Ovarian

Items 288–289

288. A 23-year-old woman returns home after delivering a healthy baby girl. She notes over the next week that she has become increasingly irritable and is not sleeping very well. She worries that she will not be a good mother and that she will make an error in caring for her baby. What is the most likely diagnosis?
a. Postpartum depression
b. Postpartum psychosis
c. Adjustment disorder
d. Postpartum blues
e. Major depression

289. What is the prevalence of the diagnosis of the woman in question #288?

a. 5%
b. 15%
c. 35%
d. 65%
e. 85%

290. A 27-year-old woman comes to a psychiatrist with the chief complaint of feeling depressed her entire life. While she states she has never been so depressed that she has been unable to function, she never feels really good for more than a week or two at a time. She has never been suicidal or psychotic, though her self-esteem is chronically low. Which of the following diagnoses is most likely?

a. Major depression
b. Adjustment disorder
c. Cyclothymia
d. Bipolar disorder
e. Dysthymia

291. A 25-year-old man comes to the psychiatrist with a chief complaint of depressed mood for 1 month. His mother, to whom he was very close, died 1 month ago, and since that time he has felt sad and has been very tearful. He has difficulty concentrating, has lost 3 lb, and is not sleeping soundly through the night. Which of the following diagnoses is most likely?

a. Major depression
b. Dysthymia
c. Posttraumatic stress disorder
d. Adjustment disorder
e. Uncomplicated bereavement

Items 292–293

292. A 32-year-old woman is brought to the emergency room by the police after she was found standing in the middle of a busy highway, naked, commanding the traffic to stop. In the emergency room she is agitated and restless, with pressured speech and an affect that alternates between euphoric and irritable. Her father is contacted and states that this kind of behavior runs in the family. Which of the following diagnoses is most likely?

a. Delirium
b. Bipolar disorder, manic
c. Bipolar disorder, mixed state
d. Cyclothymia
e. Schizophrenia

293. The resident on call decides to start the patient on a medication to control this disease. The patient refuses the medication, stating that she has taken it in the past and it causes her to be constantly thirsty and break out in pimples and makes her food taste funny. Which of the following medications is being discussed?

a. Valproic acid
b. Haloperidol
c. Carbamazepine
d. Lithium
e. Sertraline

294. A 52-year-old man comes to the physician with the chief complaint of feeling depressed for the past 2 months. He notes that he is not sleeping well, has lost 25 lb in the last 6 weeks, and is having anergia and anhedonia. In addition, in the past 4 weeks he has begun to hear the voice of his dead father telling him that he is a failure and he has begun worrying that his organs are rotting away. Which of the following statements is true?

a. The patient should be started on an SSRI and an antipsychotic
b. The patient is having an acute schizophrenic episode
c. The patient is likely suffering from a factitious disorder with psychological symptoms
d. The patient is likely abusing alcohol
e. The patient should be started on an SSRI alone

295. What is the prevalence of a clinical depression among patients post-stroke?
a. 1 to 2%
b. 10 to 15%
c. 35 to 45%
d. 75 to 80%
e. 90 to 100%

296. A 26-year-old man comes to the physician with the chief complaint of a depressed mood for the past 5 weeks. He has been feeling down, with decreased concentration, energy, and interest in his usual hobbies. Six weeks prior to this office visit he had been to the emergency room for an acute asthma attack, for which he had been started on prednisone. Which of the following diagnoses is most likely?
a. Mood disorder secondary to a general medical condition
b. Substance-induced mood disorder
c. Major depression
d. Adjustment disorder
e. Dysthymia

297. What percentage of new mothers is believed to develop postpartum depression?
a. <1%
b. 10 to 15%
c. 25 to 30%
d. 35 to 40%
e. >50%

298. How long after a stroke is a patient at a higher risk for developing a depressive disorder?
a. 2 weeks
b. 2 months
c. 6 months
d. 1 year
e. 2 years

299. A 22-year-old college student calls his psychiatrist because he notes that for the past week, after cramming hard for finals, that his thoughts have been racing and he is irritable. The psychiatrist notes that the patient's speech is pressured as well. The patient has been stable for the past 6 months on 500 milligrams of valproate twice a day. What is the first step the psychiatrist should take in the management of this patient's symptoms?
a. Hospitalize the patient
b. Increase the valproate by 500 mg/d
c. Prescribe clonazepam 1 mg qhs
d. Start haloperidol 5 mg qd
e. Tell the patient to begin psychotherapy one time per week

300. What is the lifetime risk for suicide in patients with mood disorders?
a. 1 to 3%
b. 3 to 5%
c. 10 to 15%
d. 20 to 30%
e. 30 to 40%

301. The idea that psychiatric symptoms, including a depressed mood, can result from unempathic, erratic, or neglectful parenting that prevents the development of a stable and coherent self is associated with which psychoanalyst's theory?
a. Franz Alexander
b. Carl Jung
c. Harry Stack Sullivan
d. Heinz Kohut
e. Sigmund Freud

302. A 38-year-old woman with bipolar disorder has been stable on lithium for the past 2 years. She comes to her psychiatrist's office in tears after a 2-week history of a depressed mood, poor concentration, loss of appetite, and passive suicidal ideation. Which of the following steps should the psychiatrist take next?
a. Start the patient on a second mood stabilizer
b. Start the patient on a long-acting benzodiazepine
c. Stop the lithium and start an antidepressant
d. Start an antidepressant and continue the lithium
e. Stop the lithium and start an antipsychotic

303. A 27-year-old woman has been feeling blue for the past 2 weeks. She has little energy and has trouble concentrating. She states that 6 weeks ago she had been feeling very good, with lots of energy and no need for sleep. She states this pattern has been occurring for at least the past 3 years, though the episodes have never been so severe that she couldn't work. Which of the following diagnoses is most likely?

a. Borderline personality disorder
b. Seasonal affective disorder
c. Cyclothymic disorder
d. Major depression, recurrent
e. Bipolar disorder, depressed

304. Which is the most commonly encountered psychological problem in women taking oral contraceptives?

a. Anxiety
b. Depression
c. Insomnia
d. Memory deficits
e. Illusions

DIRECTIONS: Each group of questions below consists of lettered options followed by a set of numbered items. For each numbered item, select the **one** lettered option with which it is **most** closely associated. Each lettered option may be used once, more than once, or not at all.

Items 305–309

a. Kraepelin
b. Freud
c. Bleuler
d. Beck
e. Bowlby
f. Mahler
g. Klein
h. Sullivan

305. Which analyst is most closely associated with the theory that depression is due to anger turned inward? **(CHOOSE 1 ANALYST)**

306. Which analyst is most closely associated with the theory that depression results from specific cognitive distortions present in depression-prone people? **(CHOOSE 1 ANALYST)**

307. Which analyst is most closely associated with the theory that depression is a consequence of suboptimal attachment? **(CHOOSE 1 ANALYST)**

308. Which analyst is most closely associated with the theory that depression arises from interpersonal conflict and loss of important relationships? **(CHOOSE 1 ANALYST)**

309. Which analyst is most closely associated with the theory that depression is a consequence of the reactivation of the "depressive position" from childhood? **(CHOOSE 1 ANALYST)**

310. A 42-year-old man is hospitalized after he is rescued from a rooftop where he had gone to commit suicide. He is found to have a major depression with psychotic features. Due to his severe illness and unremitting suicidal ideation, ECT is recommended. Which of the following statements is true?

a. ECT is not effective for major depression with psychosis
b. ECT should not be used unless at least three trials of antidepressants have been attempted
c. The patient should be premedicated with lorazepam before the ECT
d. ECT has a >75% change of being effective with this patient
e. The patient will need at least 25 treatments of ECT

311. A 10-year-old boy is brought to the psychiatrist by his mother. She states that for the past 2 months he has been increasingly irritable, withdrawn, and apathetic. He has been refusing to do his homework, and his grades have dropped. Which of the following statements is true?

a. The patient should be hospitalized
b. Psychotic symptoms are not found in a child so young
c. Irritability is a common mood seen in children with major depression
d. Almost all children diagnosed with depression this early end up with a diagnosis of bipolar disorder
e. The child should receive lithium and an antidepressant

312. A 35-year-old woman is seeing a psychiatrist for treatment of her major depression. After 4 weeks on fluoxetine at 40 mg/d, her psychiatrist decides to try augmentation. Which medication should the psychiatrist choose?

a. Lithium
b. Sertraline
c. An MAO inhibitor
d. Clonazepam
e. Haloperidol

313. Which of the following is a relative contraindication for ECT?

a. Space-occupying lesion in the brain
b. Pregnancy
c. Hypertension
d. Seizure disorder
e. Status post–myocardial infarction 6 months earlier

314. What is the prevalence of alcoholism among patients with a history of major depression?
a. 5%
b. 10%
c. 20%
d. 35%
e. 60%

315. A middle-aged woman presents with a variety of cognitive and somatic symptoms, fatigue, and memory loss. She denies feeling sad, but her family physician, who is aware of this patient's lifelong inability to identify and express feelings, suspects she is depressed. Which test results are more likely to confirm a diagnosis of depression?
a. Reduced metabolic activity and blood flow in both frontal lobes on PET scan
b. Diffuse cortical atrophy on CAT scan
c. Atrophy of the caudate on MRI
d. Prolonged REM sleep latency in a sleep study
e. Subcortical infarcts on MRI

316. A cognitive behavioral therapist routinely asks his depressed patients to complete a 21-item rating scale once a week to monitor changes in symptom severity. Each item in the rating scale refers to a symptom of depression, with four statements describing increasing levels of severity. Which of the following is the correct name for this rating scale, commonly used in clinical settings?
a. Minnesota Multiphasic Personality Inventory (MMPI)
b. Wechsler Adult Intelligence Scale (WAIS)
c. Thematic apperception test (TAT)
d. Beck Depression Inventory (BDI)
e. Global Assessment of Functioning Scale (GAF)

Items 317–320

Match each patient's symptoms with the most appropriate diagnosis.
a. Atypical depression
b. Double depression
c. Cyclothymic disorder
d. Melancholic depression
e. Schizoaffective disorder
f. Seasonal affective disorder

317. An elderly man has been profoundly depressed for several weeks. He cries easily and he is intensely preoccupied about trivial episodes of his past, which he considers unforgivable sins. This patient awakens every morning at 3 a.m. and cannot go back to sleep. Anything his family has tried to cheer him up has failed. He has completely lost his appetite and appears gaunt and emaciated. **(SELECT 1 DIAGNOSIS)**

318. A young woman who has felt mildly unhappy and dissatisfied with herself for most of her life has been severely depressed, irritable, and anhedonic for 3 weeks. **(SELECT 1 DIAGNOSIS)**

319. For the past 6 weeks, a middle-aged woman's mood has been mostly depressed, but she cheers up briefly when her grandchildren visit or in coincidence with other pleasant events. She is consistently less depressed in the morning than at night. When her children fail to call on the phone to inquire about her health, her mood deteriorates even more. She sleeps 14 h every night and has gained 24 lb. **(SELECT 1 DIAGNOSIS)**

320. Since he moved to Maine from his native Florida 3 years earlier, a college student has had great difficulty preparing for the winter term courses. He starts craving sweets and feeling sluggish, fatigued, and irritable in late October. These symptoms worsen gradually during the following months, and by February he has consistently gained several pounds. His mood and energy level start improving in March, and by May he is back to baseline. **(SELECT 1 DIAGNOSIS)**

Mood Disorders

Answers

286. The answer is d. (*Kaplan, 8/e, p 542–543.*) Twin studies are useful tools to separate biological and environmental etiologic factors in illnesses. Most twin studies start with the selection of monozygotic and same-sex dizygotic twin pairs who are raised together, in which one of the twins has the disorder. The other twin is then followed to determine if he or she also develops the disorder. The proportion of the twin pairs in which both twins are affected is called concordance. The difference in the concordance rate between the monozygotic and the dizygotic pairs reflects the importance of hereditary factors in the development of the disorder. The concordance rate for mood disorders in monozygotic twins averages 70% when various studies are combined. The concordance rate in dizygotic twins is approximately 20%. This is significantly higher than that found in the general population, but still 2 to 4 times lower than the concordance in monozygotic twins. These studies prove that, although environmental factors do play a role in mood disorders (the concordance is not 100%), heredity has a major role.

287. The answer is d. (*Kaplan, 8/e, p 820.*) Major depression can be the first manifestation of an occult carcinoma of the pancreas. The mechanism for this phenomenon is not known, although it may be due to humoral factors secreted by the tumor that act directly on the brain.

288–289. The answers are 288-d, 289-c. (*Kaplan, 8/e, p 27.*) Postpartum blues are very frequent, with a prevalence estimated between 20 and 40%. Symptoms include tearfulness, irritability, anxiety, and mood lability. Symptoms usually emerge during the first 2 to 4 days after birth, peak between days 5 and 7, and resolve by the end of the second week postpartum. This condition resolves spontaneously, and usually the only interventions necessary are support and reassurance.

290. The answer is e. (*Kaplan, 8/e, pp 573–578.*) Dysthymia is defined as a chronic depression that lasts at least 2 years. Usually, it begins in late adolescence or early adulthood, and sometimes patients describe being depressed for as long as they can remember. Symptoms fluctuate but are usually not severe. Patients tend to have low self-esteem and perceive themselves as inadequate and inferior to others. The somatic symptoms characteristic of major depression or melancholia are less prominent in dysthymia.

291. The answer is e. *(Kaplan, 8/e, p 558.)* The loss of a loved one is often accompanied by symptoms reminiscent of major depression, such as sadness, weepiness, insomnia, reduced appetite, and weight loss. When these symptoms do not persist beyond 2 months after the loss, they are considered a normal manifestation of bereavement. A diagnosis of major depression in these circumstances requires the presence of marked functional impairment, morbid preoccupations with unrealistic guilt or worthlessness, suicidal ideation, marked psychomotor retardation, and psychotic symptoms.

292. The answer is b. *(Kaplan, 8/e, p 533.)* Mood elevation, mood lability, irritability, expansive behavior, increased energy, decreased need for sleep, lack of insight, poor judgment, disinhibition, impulsivity, and pressured speech are characteristic symptoms of elated acute mania. In more severe cases, mood-congruent delusional ideations and hallucinations are present.

293. The answer is d. *(Kaplan, 8/e, p 572.)* Lithium is still the treatment of choice for acute mania and maintenance, although anticonvulsants such as valproate and carbamazepine have been proven effective. Newer anticonvulsants, such as gabapentin, topiramate, and lamotrigine, have also proved to have mood-stabilizing properties, although these medications have not been extensively studied yet. Weight gain, metallic taste, acne, hypothyroidism, and polyuria are common complaints with long-term lithium treatment.

294. The answer is a. *(Kaplan, 8/e, p 569.)* Psychotic depression is unlikely to improve without antipsychotic treatment. The doses of antipsychotic medications required are usually lower than those necessary to treat schizophrenia.

295. The answer is c. *(Kaplan, 8/e, p 530.)* Depression is the most common psychiatric disorder associated with cerebrovascular disease, occurring in 30 to 50% of poststroke patients. There is a higher incidence of depression among patients with left- rather than right-hemispheric lesions.

There is also an inverse correlation between the prevalence of depression and the distance of the lesion from the frontal pole, with the highest prevalence found in patients with lesions of the left frontal lobe.

296. The answer is b. *(Kaplan, 8/e, p 531.)* According to *DSM-IV* criteria, patients developing a mood disorder after using a substance (either illicit or prescribed) are diagnosed with a substance-induced mood disorder. The diagnosis of major depression cannot be made in the presence of either substance use or a general medical condition that might be the cause of the mood disorder. Prednisone is a common culprit in causing mood disorders ranging from depression to mania to psychosis.

297. The answer is b. *(Kaplan, 8/e, pp 27–28.)* Postpartum depression is relatively common, occurring in about 10 to 15% of new mothers. Symptoms are indistinguishable from those characteristic of nonpsychotic major depression and usually develop insidiously over the 6 months following delivery. Some women, however, experience an acute onset of symptoms immediately after delivery, and occasionally depression starts during pregnancy. Ambivalence toward the child and doubts about the mother's own parenting abilities are common, but the rate of suicide is low.

298. The answer is e. *(Kaplan, 8/e, p 530.)* Studies of the course and prognosis of poststroke depression indicate that the high-risk period can last up to 2 years. The presence of depression is associated with an eightfold increase in mortality risk.

299. The answer is c. *(Kaplan, 8/e, p 572.)* Sleep deprivation has an antidepressant effect in depressed patients and may trigger a manic episode in bipolar patients. The patient is not ill enough to require hospitalization. The use of a long-acting benzodiazepine will allow the patient to return to a normal sleep pattern and generally will abort the manic episode.

300. The answer is c. *(Kaplan, 8/e, p 867.)* The lifetime risk of suicide in mood disorders is between 10 and 15%. The risk is high in mania as well as depression. Patients with mixed episodes characterized by a combination of rage, depression, and grandiosity are more likely to involve others in their suicide attempts. As many as 4% of people who commit suicide murder someone else first.

301. The answer is d. (*Kaplan, 8/e, p 228.*) Heinz Kohut's theory of psychopathology focuses on intrapsychic developmental deficits, as opposed to the classical psychoanalytic view that psychiatric disorders are due to repressed drives and intrapsychic conflicts. Kohut believed that psychological health is based on a coherent, stable sense of self, which can develop only if a child receives consistent, empathic validation from his or her caretakers. When the early years are marked by emotional neglect and empathic failure, the child is left with a fragmented, unstable, and easily threatened sense of self. In adulthood, this developmental deficit manifests with low self-esteem, extreme need for others' approval, and a tendency to experience anxiety and depression whenever the already fragile self is threatened by interpersonal losses, rejection, or criticism.

302. The answer is d. (*Kaplan, 8/e, p 572.*) Since lithium and other mood stabilizers are more effective in the prevention of manic episodes than in the prevention of depression, antidepressants are used as an adjunctive treatment when depressive episodes develop during maintenance with a mood stabilizer. Since the incidence of antidepressant-induced mania is high (up to 30%), and since antidepressant treatment may cause rapid cycling, the antidepressant should be tapered and discontinued as soon as the depressive symptoms remit. Among the antidepressants in common use, buproprion is considered to carry a slightly lower risk of triggering mania.

303. The answer is c. (*Kaplan, 8/e, pp 578–580.*) Cyclothymic disorder is characterized by recurrent periods of mild depression alternating with periods of hypomania. This pattern must be present for at least 2 years (1 year for children and adolescents) before the diagnosis can be made. During these 2 years, the symptom-free intervals should not be longer than 2 months. Cyclothymic disorder usually starts during adolescence or early adulthood and tends to have a chronic course. The marked shifts in mood of cyclothymic disorder can be confused with the affective instability of borderline personality disorder or may suggest a substance abuse problem.

304. The answer is b. (*Kaplan, 8/e, p 24.*) Many studies have been done to determine the side effects of oral contraceptives, and the results are somewhat inconsistent. Most studies suggest that, although the majority of women have no significant side effects, there is an increased incidence of depression associated with this type of contraception.

305–309. The answers are 305-b, 306-d, 307-e, 308-h, 309-g. *(Kaplan, 8/e, pp 145, 206–223, 228, 562.)* In his paper "Mourning and Melancholia," Freud stressed the similarity between depression and mourning and postulated that depression is a consequence of anger triggered by a loss, real or imaginary, turned toward the self. According to Beck's cognitive model, depression is the consequence of the activation of three cognitive patterns that lead patients to view themselves, their situations, and their futures in utterly negative terms (depressive triad). Due to a negative attitude toward themselves, patients believe they are deficient, inferior, and unlovable. The second component of the depressive triad refers to the depressed patients' tendency to give a negative interpretation to everyday events and to past experiences. Finally, depressed patients believe that nothing will ever change and that they will continue to suffer indefinitely. Bowlby studied the effects of faulty attachment patterns between young children and their caregivers. He believed that separation from a primary care figure in early life leads to infant depression and to a predisposition to depression throughout life. According to the Interpersonal School of Thought founded by Sullivan, secure interpersonal relationships are essential to healthy development and to subsequent psychological stability. Sullivan theorized that conflicted relationships and loss of relationships (due to death or other changes in the environment) cause depression. Melanie Klein, who was part of the Object Relation movement, believed that depression is a consequence of the reactivation of the "depressive position," an early psychological developmental stage during which the young child experiences sadness because he or she fears having destroyed the "good object" through his or her hate and rage.

310. The answer is d. *(Kaplan, 8/e, pp 1115–1121.)* When compared to antidepressants, ECT is at least as effective and usually more effective. ECT is the recommended treatment for patients with major depression who have not responded to medications, have severe psychotic symptoms, or are highly suicidal, as well as for medically ill patients and depressed patients who cannot tolerate medications' side effects. ECT is also effective in the treatment of catatonic states and has been used to treat mania, schizophrenia, and neuroleptic malignant syndrome with variable results. ECT is particularly useful in Parkinson's disease patients with depression because it also decreases their extrapyramidal symptoms. ECT is a safe procedure with very few contraindications (recent myocardial infarcts, increased intracranial pressure, aneurysms, bleeding disorders, or any condition that disrupts the blood-brain barrier). A course of ECT treatments is typically 10 sessions long. The patient should not be given any medication (including lorazepam) that will raise the seizure threshold.

311. The answer is c. *(Kaplan, 8/e, p 553.)* Major depression is not a rare occurrence in children. Prevalence rates are 0.3% in preschoolers, 0.4 to 3% in school-age children, and 0.4 to 4.6% in adolescents. Making a correct diagnosis is complicated by the fact that the presentation of juvenile depression often differs from the adult presentation. Depressed preschoolers tend to be irritable, aggressive, withdrawn, or clingy instead of sad. In school-age children, the main manifestation of depression may be a significant loss of interest in friends and school. By adolescence, presenting symptoms of depression become more similar to those of adults. Psychotic symptoms are common in depressed children, most commonly one voice that makes depreciative comments and mood-congruent delusional ideations. Up to one-third of children diagnosed with major depression receive a diagnosis of bipolar disorder later in life. This evolution is more likely when the depressive episode has an abrupt onset and is accompanied by psychotic symptoms. Childhood depression can be treated pharmacologically, but children's response to medications differs from adult response. SSRIs have been proven effective in preschoolers and school-age children; TCAs have not. There are insufficient data about the efficacy of newer antidepressants such as nefazodone, venlafaxine, bupropion, and mirtazapine. The response of older adolescents to antidepressants is equivalent to the adult response.

312. The answer is a. *(Kaplan, 8/e, p 571.)* Lithium has been proven effective when added to an antidepressant in the treatment of refractory depression. More than one mechanism of action is probably involved, although lithium's ability to increase the presynaptic release of serotonin is the best understood. Other augmentation strategies include the use of thyroid hormones, stimulants, estrogens, and light therapy. The combination of two SSRIs (in this case fluoxetine and sertraline) or of an MAOI and an SSRI is not recommended due to the risk of precipitating a serotonin syndrome.

313. The answer is a. *(Kaplan, 8/e, pp 1115–1121.)* ECT is a safe procedure with very few contraindications (recent myocardial infarcts, increased intracranial pressure, aneurysms, bleeding disorders, and any condition that disrupts the blood-brain barrier).

314. The answer is d. *(Kaplan, 8/e, p 393.)* The prevalence of alcoholism among patients with a history of major depression sometime during their lives is 30 to 40%. The presence of alcohol abuse worsens the prognosis for both unipolar depression and bipolar disorder.

315. The answer is a. *(Kaplan, 8/e, p 542.)* Positron emission tomography (PET) scan has consistently demonstrated a decrease in blood flow and metabolism in the frontal lobe of depressed patients. Most studies have found bilateral rather than unilateral deficits and equivalent decreases in several types of depression (unipolar, bipolar, associated with OCD). Cortical atrophy and subcortical infarcts are associated, respectively, with Alzheimer's disease and multi-infarct dementia. Atrophy of the caudate is characteristic of Huntington's disease. In major depression, the REM sleep latency (the period of time between falling asleep and the first period of REM sleep) is shortened, not prolonged.

316. The answer is d. *(Ebert, pp 165–166.)* The Beck Depression Inventory is commonly used in clinical practice as a diagnostic tool and to monitor symptoms of depression during treatment. The Global Assessment of Functioning Scale (GAF) provides a measure of overall functioning in relation to the patient's psychiatric symptoms and was developed to rate Axis V of *DSM-IV*. The WAIS is used to quantify intelligence in adults. The thematic apperception test is a projective test used to explore patients' attitudes toward and expectations of themselves and others. The MMPI is used to clarify personality traits and characterological styles.

317–320. The answers are 317-d, 318-b, 319-a, 320-f. *(Kaplan, 8/e, pp 524–580.)* Melancholic depression, a variant of major depressive disorder, is characterized by loss of pleasure in all activities (anhedonia), lack of reactivity (nothing can make the patient feel better), intense guilt, significant weight loss, early morning awakening, and marked psychomotor retardation. TCAs have been considered to be more effective than other antidepressants in the treatment of melancholic depression. Double depression is diagnosed when a major depressive episode develops in a patient with dysthymic disorder. Between 68 and 90% of patients with dysthymic disorder experience at least one episode of major depression during their lives. Compared with patients who are euthymic between depressive episodes, dysthymic patients with superimposed major depression experience a higher risk for suicide, more severe depressive symptoms, more psychosocial impairment, and more treatment resistance. Atypical depression, another variant of major depressive disorder, is characterized by mood reactivity (pleasurable events may temporarily improve the mood), self-pity, excessive sensitivity to rejection, reversed diurnal mood fluctuations (patients feel better in the morning), and reversed vegetative symptoms (increased appetite and increased sleep). Approximately 15% of patients with depression have atypical features. MAOIs are considered to be more effective than other classes of antidepressants in atypical depression. Seasonal affective disorder is characterized by a regular temporal relationship between the appearance of symptoms of depression or mania and a particular time of the year. Depression characteristically starts in the fall and resolves spontaneously in spring, with a mean duration of 5 to 6 months. Characteristic symptoms include irritability, increased appetite with carbohydrate craving, increased sleep, and increased weight. The shortening of the day is the precipitant for seasonal depression. Manic episodes are associated with increased length of daylight and, consequently, with the summer months.

Anxiety, Somatoform, and Dissociative Disorders

Questions

DIRECTIONS: Each item below contains a question or incomplete statement followed by suggested responses. Select the **one best** response to each question.

321. A 23-year-old woman arrives at the emergency room complaining that, out of the blue, she had been seized by an overwhelming fear, associated with shortness of breath and a pounding heart. These symptoms lasted for approximately 20 min, and, while she was experiencing them, she feared that she was dying or going crazy. The patient has had four similar episodes during the past month, and she has been worrying that they will continue recurring. Which of the following diagnoses is most likely?

a. Acute psychotic episode
b. Hypochondriasis
c. Panic disorder
d. Generalized anxiety disorder
e. Posttraumatic stress disorder

322. A middle-aged man is chronically preoccupied with his health. For many years he feared that his irregular bowel functions meant he had cancer. Now he is very preoccupied about having a serious heart disease, despite his physician's assurance that the occasional "extra beats" he detects when he checks his pulse are completely benign. What is his most likely diagnosis?

a. Somatization disorder
b. Hypochondriasis
c. Delusional disorder
d. Pain disorder
e. Conversion disorder

193

323. After witnessing a violent argument between her parents, a young woman develops sudden blindness, but does not appear as distraught as would be expected by this development. Her pupils react normally to light, and she manages to somehow avoid obstacles when walking. Her parents, who are in the middle of a bitter divorce, put aside their differences to focus on their daughter's illness. What is the most likely diagnosis?

a. Factitious disorder
b. Malingering
c. Somatization disorder
d. Conversion disorder
e. Histrionic personality disorder

324. A college student previously in good health develops transient bladder incontinence that resolves slowly over a period of several weeks. Three months later, after breaking up with her boyfriend, she presents to her doctor's office complaining of weakness in her right leg that developed suddenly. What medical disorder, often confused with conversion disorder, is likely to have such presentation?

a. Myasthenia gravis
b. Guillain-Barré syndrome
c. Brain tumor
d. Creutzfeldt-Jakob disease
e. Multiple sclerosis

Items 325–326

325. A 28-year-old taxi driver is chronically consumed by fears of having accidentally run over a pedestrian. Although he tries to convince himself that his worries are silly, his anxiety continues to mount until he drives back to the scene of the "accident" and proves to himself that nobody lies hurt in the street. This behavior is an example of which of the following?

a. A compulsion secondary to an obsession
b. An obsession triggered by a compulsion
c. A delusional ideation
d. A typical manifestation of obsessive-compulsive personality disorder
e. A phobia

326. Which of the following statements about obsessive-compulsive disorder is correct?
a. It usually has an onset in middle age
b. It has a lifetime prevalence of 2.5%
c. It is usually caused by traumatic events
d. It is not responsive to pharmacological intervention
e. It has frequent spontaneous periods of complete remission

327. A young woman, who has a very limited memory of her childhood years but knows that she was removed from her parents due to abuse and neglect, frequently cannot account for hours or even days of her life. She hears voices that alternatively plead, reprimand, or simply comment on what she is doing. Occasionally, she does not remember how and when she arrived at a specific location. She finds clothes she does not like in her closet, and she does not remember having bought them. Her friends are puzzled because sometimes she acts in a childish, dependent way and at other times becomes uncharacteristically aggressive and controlling. These symptoms are commonly seen in which disorder?
a. Dissociative amnesia
b. Depersonalization disorder
c. Korsakoff dementia
d. Dissociative identity disorder
e. Schizophrenia

328. A 45-year-old woman was physically and sexually assaulted in her own house by two intruders. She cannot remember anything about the incident. Which of the following statements is true with regard to this type of amnesia?
a. The majority of people with this disorder also carry a variety of other serious psychiatric diagnoses
b. Most cases revert spontaneously
c. The period of memory loss is never more than a few hours
d. This disorder is very rare
e. The loss of memory is usually irreversible

329. Which of the following statements about buspirone is true?

a. It is a benzodiazepine
b. It is particularly useful for the rapid treatment of acute anxiety states
c. It is the most sedating of the commonly used antianxiety drugs
d. On a per-milligram basis, it is three times more potent than diazepam
e. It has less potential for abuse than diazepam

Items 330–331

330. A 34-year-old secretary climbs 12 flights of stairs every day to reach her office because she is terrified by the thought of being trapped in the elevator. She has never had any traumatic event occur with an elevator, but nonetheless has been terrified of them since childhood. Which of the following diagnoses is most likely?

a. Social phobia
b. Performance anxiety
c. Generalized anxiety disorder
d. Specific phobia
e. Agoraphobia

331. What is the treatment of choice for this disorder?

a. Imipramine
b. Clonazepam
c. Propanolol
d. Exposure therapy
e. Psychoanalysis

332. A 27-year-old librarian has been worried that the small lymph nodes she can palpate in her groin are a sign of lymphoma. She also worries about developing laryngeal cancer due to the second-hand smoke she is exposed to at home. For a diagnosis of hypochondriasis, her symptoms should have been present for at least what period of time?

a. 1 month
b. 3 months
c. 6 months
d. 1 year
e. 3 years

333. A young executive is periodically required to give reports of his department's progress in front of the firm's CEO. Although usually confident and well prepared, the young man becomes very anxious prior to each presentation. Once he is in front of his audience, he experiences dry mouth, heart palpitations, and profuse sweating. Which of the following statements concerning this disorder is correct?

a. Females have a higher prevalence
b. Onset in adolescence is rare
c. Medications are not effective treatment options
d. Cognitive behavioral therapy has been proved to be effective
e. Heredity does not play a role

334. During the hectic weeks preceding her wedding, a 22-year-old woman in good health and without a previous history of psychiatric illness occasionally feels unreal and detached from her own body, "like in a dream." The episodes last a few minutes and resolve spontaneously. Which of the following statements is correct?

a. These symptoms can occur in people without psychiatric disorders
b. The patient suffers from depersonalization disorder
c. Depersonalization symptoms are rare in other psychiatric disorders
d. The patient suffers from somatization disorder
e. The patient is malingering

DIRECTIONS: Each group of questions below consists of lettered options followed by a set of numbered items. For each numbered item, select the **one** lettered option with which it is **most** closely associated. Each lettered option may be used once, more than once, or not at all.

Items 335–337

Match each patient's symptoms with the most likely diagnosis.

a. Agoraphobia
b. Panic disorder
c. Obsessive-compulsive disorder
d. Social phobia
e. Adjustment disorder
f. Specific phobia
g. Acute stress disorder

335. A 45-year-old policeman who has demonstrated great courage on more than one occasion while on duty is terrified of needles. **(SELECT 1 DIAGNOSIS)**

336. For several months, a 32-year-old housewife has been unable to leave her house unaccompanied. When she tries to go out alone, she is overwhelmed by anxiety and fear that something terrible will happen to her and nobody will be there to help. **(SELECT 1 DIAGNOSIS)**

337. A 17-year-old girl blushes, stammers, and feels completely foolish when one of her classmates or a teacher asks her a question. She sits at the back of the class hoping not to be noticed because she is convinced that the other students think she is unattractive and stupid. **(SELECT 1 DIAGNOSIS)**

Items 338–342

Match each patient's symptoms with the most likely diagnosis.
a. Somatization disorder
b. Specific phobia
c. Dissociative identity disorder
d. Obsessive-compulsive disorder
e. Dissociative fugue
f. Posttraumatic stress disorder
g. Body dysmorphic disorder
h. Dysthymia

338. Two years after she was saved from her burning house, a 32-year-old woman continues to be distressed by recurrent dreams and intrusive thoughts about the event. **(SELECT 1 DIAGNOSIS)**

339. A 20-year-old student is very distressed by a small deviation of his nasal septum. He is convinced that this minor imperfection is disfiguring, although others can barely notice it. **(SELECT 1 DIAGNOSIS)**

340. A nun is found in a distant city working in a cabaret. She is unable to remember anything about her previous life. **(SELECT 1 DIAGNOSIS)**

341. A 35-year-old woman is often late to work because she must shower and dress in a very particular order or else she becomes increasingly anxious. **(SELECT 1 DIAGNOSIS)**

342. For the past 3 years, a 24-year-old college student has suffered from chronic headaches, fatigue, shortness of breath, dizziness, ringing ears, and constipation. He is incensed when his primary physician recommends a psychiatric evaluation because no organic cause for his symptoms could be found. **(SELECT 1 DIAGNOSIS)**

Items 343–347

Match the following patients' symptoms with the most appropriate pharmacological treatment:
a. Antipsychotic
b. Antianxiety agent (non-benzodiazepine)
c. Tricyclic antidepressant
d. Mood stabilizer
e. SSRI
f. Beta blocker

343. A young woman in line at a supermarket checkout suddenly experiences acute anxiety, shortness of breath, and dizziness. Her heart pounding, she runs out of the store. **(CHOOSE 1 TREATMENT)**

344. A woman washes her hands hundreds of times a day for fear of contamination. She cannot stop herself although her hands are raw and chafed. **(CHOOSE 1 TREATMENT)**

345. A Vietnam veteran startles and starts hyperventilating whenever he hears a sharp noise. **(CHOOSE 1 TREATMENT)**

346. A middle-aged bank teller with a past history of alcohol and benzodiazepine abuse, who describes himself as a chronic worrier, has been promoted to a position with increased responsibilities. Since the promotion, he has been constantly worrying about his job. He fears his superiors have made a mistake and they will soon realize he is not the right person for that position. He ruminates about unlikely future catastrophes, such as not being able to pay his bills and having to declare bankruptcy, if he is fired. He has trouble falling asleep at night and suffers from frequent headaches and acid indigestion. **(CHOOSE 2 TREATMENTS)**

347. A talented 21-year-old violinist's musical career is in jeopardy because he becomes acutely anxious whenever he is asked to play in front of an audience. **(CHOOSE 1 TREATMENT)**

Anxiety, Somatoform, and Dissociative Disorders

Answers

321. The answer is c. *(Ebert, pp 330–334.)* The patient in the question displays typical symptoms of recurrent panic attacks. Panic attacks can occur under a wide variety of psychiatric and medical conditions. The patient is diagnosed with panic disorder when there are recurrent episodes of panic and there is at least 1 month of persistent concern, worry, or behavioral change associated with the attacks. The attacks are not due to the direct effect of medical illness, medications, or substance abuse and are not better accounted for by another psychiatric disorder. While anxiety can be intense in generalized anxiety disorder, major depression, acute psychosis, and hypochondriasis, it does not have the typical presentation (i.e., a discrete episode or panic attack) described in the question.

322. The answer is b. *(Ebert, pp 371–373.)* Hypochodriasis is characterized by fear of developing or having a serious disease, based on the patient's distorted interpretation of normal physical sensations or signs. The patient continues worrying even though physical exams and diagnostic tests fail to reveal any pathological process. The fears do not have the absolute certainty of delusions. Hypochondriasis can develop in every age group, but onset is most common between 20 and 30 years of age. Both genders are equally represented, and there are no differences in prevalence based on social, educational, or marital status. The disorder tends to have a chronic, relapsing course.

323. The answer is d. *(Ebert, pp 366–369.)* Conversion disorder is characterized by the sudden appearance of one or more symptoms simulating an acute neurological illness, in the context of severe psychological stress. The symptoms with which conversion disorder manifests conform to the patient's own understanding of the medical condition and are not associated with the usual diagnostic signs. Contrary to malingering and factitious disorder, conversion disorder is nonvolitional. Conversion disorder is more frequent in women, with a female to male ratio of 2–5:1. In childhood, both sexes are equally represented. Prevalence is highest in rural areas and among the underprivileged, the undereducated, and the cognitively delayed. The sudden onset and the temporal relation to a severe stress help differentiate conversion disorder from more chronic conditions such as somatization disorder and personality disorders.

324. The answer is e. *(Ebert, p 368.)* Many serious neurological disorders can be mistaken for conversion disorder. The differential diagnosis can be particularly challenging with multiple sclerosis, a disorder also characterized by the sudden appearance of neurological symptoms that, at least in the beginning, often resolve spontaneously. Other causes of possible diagnostic confusion are the fact that symptoms in multiple sclerosis may be precipitated by stress and that multiple sclerosis, like conversion disorder, is more frequent in women.

325. The answer is a. *(Ebert, pp 353–354.)* Recurrent obsessions and compulsions are essential features of obsessive-compulsive disorder (OCD). Obsessions are persistent thoughts or mental images that are subjectively experienced as intrusive and alien and characteristically provoke various levels of anxiety. Compulsions are repetitive acts, behaviors, or thoughts designed to counteract the anxiety elicited by the obsessions. The diagnosis of obsessive-compulsive personality disorder is reserved for those patients with significant impairments in their occupational or social effectiveness. These patients are preoccupied with rules, regulations, orderliness, neatness, details, and the achievement of perfection.

326. The answer is b. *(Ebert, p 352.)* Obsessive-compulsive disorder usually has its onset from late childhood to early adulthood and has a lifetime prevalence of about 2.5%. Stress is usually associated with worsening of symptoms, but traumatic events do not cause this disorder. While a minority of patients do have periods of complete remission, about one-third have a fluctuating course and up to 60% have a constant or progressive course. Many patients are markedly improved by pharmacological intervention. The most commonly used agents are serotonin reuptake inhibitors such as fluoxetine and sertraline, although the tricyclic clomipramine is also used.

Anxiety, Somatoform, and Dissociative Disorders   *Answers*   **203**

327. The answer is d. *(Ebert, pp 388–391.)* Losing time and memory gaps, including significant gaps in autobiographical memory, are typical symptoms of dissociative identity disorder (previously known as multiple personality disorder). Patients also report fluctuation in their skills, well-learned abilities, and habits. This is explained as a state-dependent disturbance of implicit memory. Hallucinations in all sensory modalities are common. Dramatic changes in mannerisms, tone of voice, and affect are manifestations of this disorder.

328. The answer is b. *(Ebert, pp 387–388.)* Dissociative amnesia is the inability to recall important personal information, usually of a traumatic nature, which cannot be explained by ordinary forgetfulness. Dissociative amnesia is the most common of all dissociative disorders and is most frequent in the third and fourth decades of life. Although a minority of patients present with a comorbid diagnosis (other dissociative disorders, alcohol abuse, depression, personality disorders), most patients with dissociative amnesia do not have other significant psychiatric history. The memory loss can extend from minutes to years. Most cases of dissociative amnesia resolve spontaneously, usually after the stressful situation is removed and the individual feels safe. In cases that do not resolve spontaneously, hypnosis and interviews aided by medications (benzodiazepines and barbiturates) are used.

329. The answer is e. *(Ebert, p 339.)* Buspirone and benzodiazepines have different chemical structures. Buspirone's potency is equivalent to the potency of diazepam. Since it takes approximately 3 weeks for the antianxiety effects to appear, buspirone is not useful for anxiety conditions that require acute intervention. Buspirone is less sedating than benzodiazepines and appears to have less potential for abuse.

330. The answer is d. *(Ebert, pp 334–337.)* Specific phobias are characterized by an unreasonable or excessive fear of an object, an animal, or a situation (flying, being trapped in close spaces, heights, blood, spiders, etc.). Since the exposure to the feared situation, animal, or object causes an immediate surge of anxiety, patients carefully avoid the phobic stimuli. The diagnosis of specific phobia requires the presence of reduced functioning and interference with social activities and relationships due to the avoidant behavior, anticipatory anxiety, and distress caused by the exposure to the feared stimulus. In social phobias and performance anxiety, patients fear social interactions (in general or limited to specific situations) and public performance (public speaking, acting, playing an instrument), respectively. In generalized anxiety disorder, the anxiety is more chronic and less intense than in a phobic disorder and is not limited to a specific situation or item. Agoraphobic patients fear places where escape may be difficult or help may not be available in case the patient has a panic attack. Agoraphobic patients are often prisoners in their own homes and depend on a companion when they need to go out.

331. The answer is d. *(Ebert, pp 336–337.)* No medication has proved to be effective in treating specific phobias. The treatment of choice in specific phobias is exposure, in vivo or using techniques of guided imagery, pairing relaxation exercises with exposure to the feared stimulus. The patient can be exposed to the feared stimulus gradually or can be asked to immediately confront the most anxiety-provoking situation (flooding).

332. The answer is c. *(Ebert, p 371.)* Hypochondriasis is defined by *DSM-IV* as a persistent fear, despite medical reassurance, that one has a serious physical illness. The patient's beliefs are based on misinterpretation of benign bodily symptoms. The belief is not of delusional proportions, and the condition must persist for 6 months for this diagnosis to be made. It is estimated that from 3 to 14% of patients seen in a general medical practice may suffer from hypochondriasis.

333. The answer is d. *(Ebert, pp 334–337.)* The patient in the question suffers from social phobia triggered by public speaking. Three major cognitive behavioral techniques, usually used in combination, have been proved to be effective in the treatment of this disorder: exposure, cognitive restructuring, and social skills training. Onset of social phobia is usually during adolescence or the early adult years. Several classes of medications have also been proven effective in the treatment of social phobia, including MAO inhibitors, SSRIs, benzodiazepines, and beta blockers. Buspirone can be useful when social phobia and generalized anxiety disorder are comorbid.

334. The answer is a. *(Kaplan, 8/e, p 672.)* Occasional depersonalization experiences are common in normal adults and children, especially when under stress. To meet the diagnostic criteria for depersonalization disorder, the experiences must be persistent and severe enough to cause distress. Symptoms of depersonalization are common in a variety of psychiatric disorders including other dissociative disorders, anxiety disorders, psychotic disorders, and depression.

335–337. The answers are 335-f, 336-a, 337-d. *(Ebert, pp 330–337.)* Phobic disorders include agoraphobia, specific phobias, and social phobia. They are all characterized by overwhelming, persistent, and irrational fears that result in the overpowering need to avoid the object or situation that is generating the anxiety. Agoraphobia is the marked fear and avoidance of being alone in public places where rapid exit would be difficult or help would not be available. Social phobia is characterized by avoidance of situations in which one is exposed to scrutiny by others and by fears of being humiliated or embarrassed by one's actions. Specific phobias are triggered by objects (often animals), heights, or closed spaces. A large variety of objects are associated with simple phobias.

338–342. The answers are 338-f, 339-g, 340-e, 341-d, 342-a. *(Ebert, pp 307–311, 334–337, 341–349, 351–365, 369–371, 373–374, 387–391.)* One of the most characteristic features of posttraumatic stress disorder (PTSD) is the occurrence of repeated dreams, flashbacks, and intrusive thoughts of the traumatic event. Hyperarousal, irritability, difficulties concentrating, exaggerated startle response, emotional numbing, avoidance of places and situations associated with the traumatic experience, dissociative amnesia, and a sense of foreshortened future are other symptoms displayed by patients with PTSD. In body dysmorphic disorder, a person of normal appearance is preoccupied with some imaginary physical defect. The belief is tenacious and sometimes of delusional intensity. This diagnosis should not be made when the distorted ideations are limited to the belief of being fat in anorexia nervosa or are limited to uneasiness with one's gender characteristics in gender identity disorder. Patients with obsessive-compulsive disorder (OCD) experience persistent thoughts, impulses, or repetitive behaviors that they are unable to stop voluntarily. Obsessions and compulsions are experienced as alien and ego-dystonic and are the source of much distress. Somatization disorder is characterized by a history of multiple physical complaints not explained by organic factors. The diagnosis requires the presence of four pain symptoms, two gastrointestinal symptoms, one sexual symptom, and one pseudoneurological symptom over the course of the disorder. The essential feature of dissociative fugue is sudden travel away from home accompanied by temporary loss of autobiographic memory. Patients are confused about their identity and at times form new identities. Dissociative fugue may last from hours to months. During the fugue, individuals do not appear to have any psychopathology; usually they come to attention when their identity is questioned.

343–347. The answers are 343-e, 344-e, 345-f, 346-b,e, 347-f. *(Ebert, pp 330–340, 345–347, 361–364.)* The young woman in the supermarket suffers from panic disorder, which responds to a variety of psychotropic medications, including SSRIs, tricyclic antidepressants, and benzodiazepines. Given the abuse potential of benzodiazepines and the significant side effects of the tricyclics, however, SSRIs are the treatment of choice for panic disorder today. Panic disorder is also treated with MAO inhibitors, although due to the risk of hypertensive crises triggered by tyramine-rich foods, these medications are not usually used as a first-line treatment. The patient with compulsive hand washing has obsessive-compulsive disorder (OCD), and she would respond to an SSRI. Treatment of OCD symptoms may require higher dosages and longer trial periods than recommended for depression. Before a trial is considered ineffective, the patient should have received minimum daily doses of sertraline 200 mg, fluoxetine 60 mg, fluvoxamine 300 mg, paroxetine 60 mg, and/or clomipramine 250 mg, since this disorder often requires higher doses than what would be seen if a major depression were being treated with the same medication. Each drug trial should be no less than 12 weeks. The Vietnam veteran's symptoms of autonomic hyperarousal are likely to respond to medications that inhibit adrenergic activity, such as beta blockers. The bank teller presents with symptoms of generalized anxiety disorder (GAD). Tricyclics, SSRIs, and buspirone (a nonbenzodiazepine antianxiolytic) are all effective in GAD, but due to the significant side effects of tricyclics, buspirone or SSRIs are most commonly used. Benzodiazepines are also very effective in this disorder, but, since they may be addictive, they are not recommended for people with a history of substance abuse. β-adrenergic receptor antagonists (beta blockers) are effective in the treatment of specific forms of social phobias such as fear of public speaking and fear of performing in front of an audience.

Personality Disorders, Human Sexuality, and Miscellaneous Syndromes

Questions

DIRECTIONS: Each item below contains a question or incomplete statement followed by suggested responses. Select the **one best** response to each question.

348. A middle-aged man with a master's degree in chemistry lives alone in a halfway house and subsists on panhandling and collecting redeemable cans. He spends most of his money on keno tickets. Ten years ago he lost his job in a large firm because he had stolen company money to bet on horses. Afterward, he had several other jobs, all short-lived because he spent more time at the track than on the job. To support his gambling habit, he borrowed large sums of money from friends and relatives, which he never repaid. Under which category is this disorder classified?

a. Personality disorders
b. Anxiety disorders
c. Impulse control disorders
d. Dissociative disorders
e. Factitious disorders

349. A 7-year-old girl gets up at night and, still asleep, walks around the house for a few minutes before returning to bed. When she is forced to awaken during one of these episodes, she is confused and disoriented. Which of the following statements about this disorder is correct?

a. Violent outbursts are possible when the individual is suddenly awakened
b. This behavior usually takes place during early morning hours
c. This behavior coincides with periods of REM sleep
d. This behavior is more common between ages 10 and 15
e. With some effort, the particulars of the previous night's episodes can be remembered the next day

350. A 65-year-old woman lives alone in a dilapidated house, although her family members have tried in vain to move her to a better dwelling. She wears odd and out-of-fashion clothes and rummages in the garbage cans of her neighbors to look for redeemable cans and bottles. She is very suspicious of her neighbors. She was convinced that her neighbors were plotting against her life for a brief time after she was mugged and thrown onto the pavement by a teenager, but now thinks that this is not the case. She believes in the "power of crystals to protect me" and has them strewn haphazardly throughout her house. What is the most likely diagnosis?

a. Autism
b. Schizophrenia, paranoid type
c. Schizotypal personality disorder
d. Avoidant personality disorder
e. Schizoid personality disorder

351. In narcolepsy, the polysomnographic recording typically shows which of the following patterns?

a. REM intrusion during inappropriate periods
b. An absence of REM sleep in midcycle
c. Spike-and-wave EEG recording
d. Extreme muscular relaxation
e. Decreased REM sleep density

352. A 24-year-old woman is chronically sleepy and fatigued. Her sleep is constantly interrupted because, as soon as she begins to fall asleep, an uncomfortable crawling feeling in her calves forces her to walk or move her legs. Which of the following conditions is often associated with this disorder?

a. Niacin deficiency
b. Panic disorder
c. Arteriosclerosis
d. Pregnancy
e. Obstructive apnea

353. An attractive and well-dressed 22-year-old woman is arrested for prostitution, but on being booked at the jail, she is found to actually be a male. The patient tells the consulting physician that he is a female trapped in a male body and he has felt that way since he was a child. He has been taking female hormones and is attempting to find a surgeon who would remove his male genitals and create a vagina. Which of the following is the most likely diagnosis?
a. Homosexuality
b. Gender identity disorder
c. Transvestite fetishism
d. Delusional disorder
e. Schizophrenia

354. Which of the following statements is true with regard to personality disorders?
a. They are minor disturbances that respond quickly to treatment
b. They cause little impairment in adaptive functioning
c. They rarely cause any subjective distress
d. They are usually evident by adolescence
e. They often have periods of remission of up to 1 year

355. Every 4 or 5 weeks, a usually well-functioning and mild-mannered 35-year-old woman experiences a few days of irritability, tearfulness, and unexplained sadness. During these days, she also feels fatigued and bloated and eats large quantities of sweets. What is the most appropriate diagnosis?
a. Cyclothymia
b. Borderline personality disorder
c. Dissociative identity disorder
d. Premenstrual dysphoric disorder
e. Minor depressive disorder

356. A 65-year-old retired steelworker who has never had any sexual dysfunction experiences difficulty in obtaining and maintaining an erection shortly after he starts taking a medication prescribed by his primary care physician. Which of the following medications is most likely to cause such a side effect?

a. Propranolol
b. Amoxicillin
c. Lorazepam
d. Bupropion
e. Thyroid hormones

357. According to *DSM-IV,* the diagnosis of an adjustment disorder is limited to which patients?

a. Those whose symptoms are in response to an identifiable stressor that occurred within the past 2 years
b. Those who do not have social impairment due to their symptoms
c. Those whose symptoms are an exacerbation of a preexisting Axis II disorder
d. Those whose distress is in excess of what would be expected as a result of the stressor
e. Those whose symptoms persist for at least 1 year after the termination of the stressor

Items 358–359

358. A demanding 25-year-old woman begins psychotherapy stating she is both desperate and bored. She reports that for the past 5 or 6 years she has experienced periodic anxiety and depression and has made several suicidal gestures. She also reports a variety of impulsive and self-defeating behaviors and sexual promiscuity. She wonders if she might be a lesbian, though most of her sexual experiences have been with men. She has abruptly terminated two previous attempts at psychotherapy. In both cases she was enraged at the therapist because he was unwilling to prescribe anxiolytic medications. Which of the following is the most likely diagnosis?

a. Dysthymia
b. Histrionic personality disorder
c. Antisocial personality disorder
d. Borderline personality disorder
e. Impulse control disorder not otherwise specified

359. A common finding in the past history of patients with this diagnosis is which of the following?

a. Childhood sexual abuse
b. Criminal activity before age 10
c. Extreme shyness
d. Compulsive orderliness
e. Persistent magical and other odd beliefs

DIRECTIONS: Each group of questions below consists of lettered options followed by a set of numbered items. For each numbered item, select the **one** lettered option with which it is **most** closely associated. Each lettered option may be used once, more than once, or not at all.

Items 360–363

Match each patient's behavior with the most appropriate personality disorder.

a. Paranoid
b. Schizotypal
c. Schizoid
d. Narcissistic
e. Borderline
f. Histrionic
g. Antisocial
h. Obsessive-compulsive
i. Dependent
j. Avoidant

360. A 28-year-old woman begins seeing a psychiatrist because "I am just so very lonely." Her speech is excessively impressionistic and lacks specific detail. She flirts constantly with the physician and is "hurt" when the therapist does not notice her new clothes or hairstyle. **(CHOOSE 1 DISORDER)**

361. A 42-year-old man comes to the psychiatrist at the insistence of his boss because he constantly misses important deadlines. The man states everyone at work is lazy and does not live up to his own standards for perfection. He is angry when the physician starts the interview 3 minutes later than the appointed time. **(CHOOSE 1 DISORDER)**

362. A 34-year-old woman comes to the psychiatrist on the advice of her mother, because the patient still lives at home and will not make any decisions without her mother's reassurance. The patient's mother accompanies the patient to the appointment. She states the patient becomes anxious when her mother must leave the home because the patient is terrified that her mother will die and the patient will have to take care of herself, something she feels incapable of doing. **(CHOOSE 1 DISORDER)**

363. A 25-year-old high school dropout has been arrested over 12 times for various assault, fraud, and attempted murder charges. He has been in many physical fights, usually after he got caught cheating at cards. On examination he seems relaxed and even cocky, and he shows no remorse for his actions. **(CHOOSE 1 DISORDER)**

364. A woman confides to her friends that for the past 3 years her husband has practically ceased to be interested in sex. Unless she solicits it, they go without sex for months. He is distressed and ashamed by his "deficiency," but nothing they have tried so far seems to rekindle his sexual desire. When he does engage in intercourse, he has no difficulty reaching and maintaining an erection or reaching an orgasm. Which of the following diagnosis is this patient most likely to have?
a. Sexual aversion disorder
b. Male erectile disorder
c. Hypoactive sexual disorder
d. Male homosexuality
e. Normal variance of sexual desire

365. Estimates of the lifetime prevalence rates of all personality disorders in the general population are in what range?
a. 0 to 1%
b. 1 to 2%
c. 3 to 5%
d. 10 to 20%
e. 20 to 30%

Items 366–367

366. A 33-year-old married man who suffers from chronic anxiety presents for a psychiatric consultation. He reports that his marriage is very happy and gives a sexual history that includes daily and satisfying sexual intercourse with his wife. He also masturbates three to four times weekly. He states that his sexual drive has been high ever since he was a teenager. His sexual fantasies are predominantly heterosexual, but occasionally he fantasizes about homosexual encounters while masturbating. During his adult years, while traveling alone, he has had both heterosexual and homosexual experiences on several occasions. He remembers these experiences as pleasurable. The patient admits to some transient guilt about "stepping out" on his wife, but he is not excessively anxious or troubled about his sexual life. On the basis of the patient's sexual history, one could reasonably infer a diagnosis of which of the following?

a. Schizotypal personality disorder
b. Antisocial personality disorder
c. Narcissistic personality disorder
d. Borderline personality disorder
e. No personality disorder

367. Which of the following statements is most likely to be true given the history of occasional homosexual fantasies and several adult homosexual experiences in a man with a background of predominantly heterosexual behavior?

a. The patient is a repressed homosexual
b. The absence of anxiety or concern about his sexuality suggests psychopathology
c. He may be bisexual, but nothing in the history suggests sexual psychopathology
d. There is a need for psychoanalysis
e. The patient has gender identity disorder

368. Which of the following statements is true with regard to patients who have paranoid personality disorder?

a. They usually also suffer from paranoid psychosis
b. They have a predisposition to develop schizophrenia
c. They often have a preoccupation with helping the weak and the powerless
d. They usually present themselves in a quiet and humble fashion
e. They are often litigious

369. Which of the following statements regarding vaginismus is true?
a. It involves the outer one-third of the vagina
b. It occurs only during attempted intercourse
c. It is initiated by erotic arousal
d. It makes female masturbation difficult
e. It is under voluntary control

Items 370–371

370. A young librarian has been exceedingly shy and fearful of people since childhood. She longs to make friends, but even casual social interactions cause her a great deal of shame and anxiety. She has never been at a party, and she has requested to work in the least active section of her library, even though this means lower pay. She cannot look at her rare customers without blushing, and she is convinced that they see her as incompetent and clumsy. Which of the following personality disorders is most likely?
a. Schizotypal
b. Avoidant
c. Dependent
d. Schizoid
e. Paranoid

371. Which anxiety disorder is most likely to be confused with this personality disorder?
a. Generalized anxiety disorder
b. Specific phobia
c. Agoraphobia
d. Social phobia
e. Obsessive compulsive disorder

372. Which of the following statements about transvestic fetishism is true?
a. Affected individuals identify themselves as members of the opposite sex and long for a sex change
b. Affected individuals are almost always male homosexuals
c. Males and females are equally represented
d. Affected individuals are aroused when dressed as a woman
e. The disorder rarely starts in childhood

Items 373–374

373. A 48-year-old male has been unable to have intercourse with his wife of 20 years since she disclosed to him that she was having an affair with his younger and more attractive work partner. He continues having spontaneous nocturnal erections. This patient's sexual dysfunction is most likely due to which of the following?

a. An organic disorder
b. A psychogenic determinant
c. A form of paraphilia
d. An irreversible psychodynamic process
e. A sexual identity disorder

374. Which of the following statements is true with regard to nocturnal erections?

a. They are usually a symptom of a psychiatric disorder
b. They take place during non-REM sleep
c. They can be decreased or absent in depression
d. They take place in the first third of the night
e. They are monitored during polysomnographic studies

375. A young woman presents to the emergency room vomiting bright red blood. Once she is medically stable, the intern who performs her physical exam notices that the enamel of her front teeth is badly eroded and her parotid glands are swollen. These medical complications are due to which of the following?

a. Inadequate caloric intake
b. Purging
c. Laxative abuse
d. Diuretic abuse
e. Ipecac toxicity

Items 376–377

376. An off-Broadway actor consistently bores his friends and acquaintances by talking incessantly about his exceptional talent and his success on the stage. He does not seem to realize that other people do not share his high opinion of his acting talent and are not interested in his monologues. When a director criticizes the way he delivers his lines during rehearsal, the actor goes into a rage and accuses the director of trying to jeopardize his career out of jealousy. Which personality disorder represents the most correct diagnosis?

a. Histrionic
b. Narcissistic
c. Borderline
d. Paranoid
e. Antisocial

377. Choose the correct statement about this personality disorder.

a. Individuals with this disorder have an unusually high self-esteem
b. Its prevalence is 5% in the general population
c. Females are more commonly affected than males
d. Symptoms tend to decrease with aging
e. Although narcissistic traits are common in adolescents, only a small minority develop a personality disorder later on

378. Which of the following statements is true with regard to factitious disorder?

a. It is synonymous with malingering
b. The patient's goal is to assume and maintain the sick role
c. The patient's goal is to avoid unpleasant consequences or work
d. Patients visit their PCP's office often but rarely are hospitalized
e. It is easily diagnosed

379. A 3-year-old girl's preferred make-believe game is playing house with her dolls. She loves to experiment with her mother's makeup and states that, when she grows up, she will be a mommy. She is very offended when someone mistakes her for a boy. This scenario demonstrates that which of the following is well established at this girl's age?

a. Theory of the mind
b. Sexual orientation
c. Gender identity
d. Gender neurosis
e. Gender dysphoria

Items 380–383

Match each patient's symptoms with the correct diagnosis.

a. Primary hypersomnia
b. Narcolepsy
c. Sleep terror disorder
d. Circadian sleep disorder
e. Primary insomnia
f. Periodic limb movement disorder
g. Sleep apnea
h. Restless legs syndrome

380. A woman complains about her husband moving his legs constantly while he sleeps. She ends up being kicked several times every night. The husband has no memory of this nighttime activity but he reports that he wakes up tired every morning despite getting what he considers an adequate amount of sleep (7 to 8 h per night). **(CHOOSE 1 DIAGNOSIS)**

381. Due to her job's requirements, a per diem nurse works different shifts almost every week. She is constantly sleepy and fatigued. However, even when she has days off, she has great difficulty falling asleep at night and remaining asleep for more than 2 to 3 h at a time. **(CHOOSE 1 DIAGNOSIS)**

382. For the past 2 years a 28-year-old man has found himself in many dangerous or embarrassing situations due to his inconvenient habit of falling abruptly asleep in the middle of any activity. Once he hit a pole because he fell asleep while driving. His wife still teases him for "taking a nap" while they are having sex. The man reports that he starts dreaming as soon as his eyes close, and, when he wakes up, 10 to 20 min later, he feels wide awake and refreshed. **(CHOOSE 1 DIAGNOSIS)**

383. A young man has felt consistently sleepy during the day for as long as he can remember. Although he sleeps from 9 to 11 h every night, he wakes up unrefreshed and needs to take naps at least once a day in order to function. According to his wife and bed partner, he does not snore and he does not kick her while sleeping. Aside from the difficulties caused by his chronic sleepiness, his history is unremarkable. **(CHOOSE 1 DIAGNOSIS)**

Items 384–387

Match each paraphilia with the appropriate presentation.

a. Frotteurism
b. Sexual sadism
c. Transvestic fetishism
d. Fetishism
e. Exhibitionism
f. Sexual masochism
g. Pedophilia
h. Paraphilia not otherwise specified

384. The career of a prominent political figure is destroyed after it becomes common knowledge that for many years he has been making obscene phone calls to young women in his neighborhood. **(CHOOSE 1 PRESENTATION)**

385. For several years, a 21-year-old male has masturbated while fantasizing about exposing his genitals to a female stranger. For a long time, fear of being arrested has kept him from acting out his fantasies, but recently he has not been able to resist the urge to expose himself to unsuspecting females. **(CHOOSE 1 PRESENTATION)**

386. A young male becomes very aroused when he rubs himself against the buttocks of young women in crowded subways at rush hour. **(CHOOSE 1 PRESENTATION)**

387. A man can become sexually aroused and can reach an orgasm only when he holds a pair of women's lacy underwear. **(CHOOSE 1 PRESENTATION)**

Personality Disorders, Human Sexuality, and Miscellaneous Syndromes

Answers

348. The answer is c. *(Ebert, pp 456–457.)* Pathological gambling is found in the diagnostic category called impulse control disorders, together with pyromania, intermittent explosive disorder, trichotillomania, kleptomania, and impulse control disorder not otherwise specified. The *DSM-IV* criteria for pathological gambling are quite similar to the criteria for substance abuse disorders: preoccupation with gambling; need to gamble increasing amounts of money to obtain the same effects; unsuccessful efforts to stop or cut back; using gambling to escape problems or relieve dysphoric mood; after money losses, returning to gambling the next day to "break even"; lying to family and friends to conceal losses and the extent of the involvement in gambling; committing illegal acts to finance the habit; and jeopardizing important relationships or losing jobs because of gambling. The vast majority of compulsive gamblers are men. The prevalence is estimated to be 0.2 to 3% of the general population, varying with the number of gaming venues available.

349. The answer is a. *(Ebert, p 443.)* Sleepwalking disorder is a parasomnia associated with slow-wave sleep. The patient is usually difficult to awaken, confused, and amnesic for the episode. Common in children, sleepwalking peaks between ages 4 and 8 years and usually disappears after adolescence. The person attempting to awaken the sleepwalker may be violently attacked. The severity of the disorder ranges from less than one episode per month without any problem to nightly episodes complicated by physical injury to the patient and others.

350. The answer is c. *(Ebert, pp 472–474.)* Schizotypal personality disorder, a cluster A disorder, is characterized by acute discomfort in close relationships, cognitive and perceptual distortions, and eccentric behavior beginning in early adulthood and present in a variety of contexts. Individuals with schizoid personality disorder do not present with the magical thinking, oddity, unusual perceptions, and odd appearance typical of schizotypal individuals. In schizophrenia, psychotic symptoms are much more prolonged and severe. Avoidant individuals avoid social interaction out of shyness and fear of rejection and not out of disinterest or suspiciousness. In autism, social interactions are more severely impaired and stereotyped behaviors are usually present.

351. The answer is a. *(Ebert, p 441.)* In narcolepsy, REM periods are not segregated in their usual rhythm during sleep, but suddenly and repeatedly intrude into wakefulness. Nocturnal sleep shows a sleep-onset REM period or one that occurs very shortly after the onset of sleep. Fifteen to 30% of patients also show some nocturnal myoclonus or sleep apnea.

352. The answer is d. *(Ebert, pp 438–439.)* The woman in the vignette suffers from restless legs syndrome, a disorder characterized by the irresistible urge to move one's legs while trying to fall asleep. Patients describe the unpleasant sensations in their calves as feeling like worms or ants crawling. Only moving the legs or walking alleviates the discomfort. Restless legs syndrome can be caused by pregnancy, anemia, renal failure, or various metabolic disorders.

353. The answer is b. *(Ebert, pp 584–586.)* In adolescents and young adults, gender identity disorder is characterized by a strong cross-gender identification, a persistent discomfort with one's sex, and clinically significant distress or impairment. Such patients usually trace their conviction to early childhood, often live as the opposite sex, and seek sex reassignment surgery and endocrine treatment. These patients feel a sense of relief and appropriateness when they are wearing opposite-sex clothing. In contrast, patients with transvestic fetishism are sexually aroused by this behavior. Homosexuality is not a diagnosis in *DSM-IV*. While some homosexuals cross-dress to seek a same-sex partner, they do not feel that they belong to the opposite sex, nor do they seek sex reassignment surgery.

354. The answer is d. *(Ebert, p 467.)* Personality disorders are characterized as deeply ingrained, inflexible, dysfunctional patterns of perceiving, thinking about, and relating to the world. Personality disorders typically cause conflicted relationships as well as general impairment of adaptive functioning. The pervasive personality traits characteristic of a personality disorder are generally recognizable by adolescence or even earlier, and they typically persist throughout most of adult life.

355. The answer is d. *(Kaplan, pp 808–809.)* The physical and emotional symptoms of premenstrual dysphoric disorder (PMDD) are restricted to the late luteal phase of the menstrual cycle and resolve 1 or 2 days after the onset of the menstruation. Although most women of childbearing age experience some symptoms of PMDD during some of their menstrual cycles, only 5 to 9% meet the criteria for the diagnosis.

356. The answer is a. *(Kaplan, p 977.)* Among beta blockers, propranolol is the most likely to cause impotence. Furthermore, through its effect on the serotonin system, propranolol can also inhibit orgasm and reduce sex drive. Fatigue and depressed mood—also frequent side effects of propranolol—can also have a negative effect on sexual function.

357. The answer is d. *(Ebert, p 460.)* According to *DSM-IV*, patients with adjustment disorders develop clinically significant symptoms in response to an identifiable psychosocial stressor. Symptoms must develop within 3 months of the onset of the stressor, and they have to be either significantly in excess of what could be normally expected in similar circumstances or cause considerable limitations in functioning. Once the stressor has terminated, the symptoms do not last longer than 6 months.

358. The answer is d. *(Ebert, pp 475–477.)* The patient's history and presenting symptoms are classic for the diagnosis of borderline personality disorder. Patients with borderline personalities present with a history of a pervasive instability of mood, relationships, and self-image beginning by early adulthood. Their behavior is often impulsive and self-damaging; their sexuality is chaotic; sexual orientation may be uncertain; and anger is intense and often acted out. Recurrent suicidal gestures are common. The shifts of mood usually last from a few hours to a few days. Patients often describe chronic feelings of boredom and emptiness.

359. The answer is a. *(Ebert, pp 475–477.)* Psychoanalytic theories have connected borderline personality disorder with a maternal inability to tolerate and encourage the 2- to 3-year-old child's efforts to become autonomous and a lack of empathy and understanding for the child's emotions. A considerable body of research has also documented a high frequency of neglect, abandonment, physical abuse, and sexual abuse in the history of individuals with this disorder.

360–363. The answers are 360-f, 361-h, 362-i, 363-g. *(Ebert, pp 474–475, 477–479, 481–484.)* Histrionic personality disorder is characterized by a chronic pattern of excessive emotionality and attention seeking. Patients with this disorder like to be the center of attention, and interaction with others is often inappropriately seductive. These patients may also use their physical appearance to draw attention to themselves. Speech is dramatic but superficial, and details are lacking. Patients are easily suggestible and influenced by others. Patients with obsessive-compulsive personality disorder are preoccupied with orderliness, perfection, and control. They are often so preoccupied with details, lists and order that they lose the forest for the trees. Their concern with perfectionism makes it difficult for them to complete projects in a timely manner. They are often perceived as rigid and stubborn. Patients with dependent personality disorder have a chronic and excessive need to be taken care of. This leads to submissive, clinging behavior in a desperate attempt to avoid being separated from the caretaker. These patients have difficulty making everyday decisions on their own, and often need considerable reassurance before being able to do so. They are also unrealistically preoccupied with fears of being left alone to take care of themselves. Individuals with antisocial personality disorder display a chronic pattern of disregard for the rights of others, and often violate them. They also are frequently irritable and aggressive, engaging in repeated physical assaults. They do not show remorse for their activities. This diagnosis is not made if the episodes of antisocial behavior are made exclusively during the course of schizophrenia or a manic episode.

364. The answer is c. *(Ebert, pp 395–397.)* Hypoactive sexual disorder is characterized by a lack of sexual desire and a frequency of sexual activity clearly lower than expected for age and context. Patients have few or no sexual fantasies, lack awareness for sexual cues, and have little interest in initiating sexual experiences. Once they are involved in a sexual act, though, they function normally. Lack of desire may be due to chronic stress, prolonged abstinence, anxiety, or unconscious fear of sex or may be a sign of a deteriorating relationship. Hypoactive sexual disorder often starts during adolescence and may last a lifetime.

365. The answer is d. *(Ebert, pp 467–468.)* Personality disorders are quite common in the general population. There is fairly good agreement that the lifetime prevalence rate of all personality disorders in the general population ranges from 5 to 20%, depending on the severity of impairment required for the diagnosis. There is less agreement about prevalence rates for specific personality disorders, largely because of sampling differences between various studies. The rate is even higher in clinical settings, with as many as 50% of psychiatric patients meeting Axis II criteria for at least one personality disorder.

366. The answer is e. *(Ebert, pp 468–469.)* There is nothing in the patient's history to suggest the presence of a personality disorder. The hallmark of a personality disorder is the presence of a constellation of behaviors or traits that cause significant impairment in social or occupational functioning or cause subjective distress. The patient in the question, on the contrary, reports a happy marriage and an ability to function well in social and occupational circumstances. While some persons in our society might object to his sexual behavior on moral grounds, such judgments are not a part of the diagnostic process.

367. The answer is c. *(Ebert, p 394.)* Sexual behavior and fantasies range on a continuum, from exclusively heterosexual to exclusively homosexual. There are many men who are predominantly heterosexual but who have engaged in homosexual behavior or have occasional homosexual fantasies, and there are many predominantly homosexual men with the capacity for heterosexual arousal. The presence of homosexual desire or behavior is not considered a sexual disorder according to the diagnostic definitions of the American Psychiatric Association. While further therapeutic inquiry may uncover sexual conflict or marital discord, the history provided does not necessarily suggest that will be the case.

368. The answer is e. *(Ebert, pp 470–471.)* Persons with a paranoid personality disorder characteristically show marked suspiciousness of others and are extremely sensitive to any potential threat or injustice. They frequently look for hidden motives or meanings, are contemptuous of the weak, and are very sensitive to issues of power and dominance. They often are moralistic or self-righteous and may be quite litigious. The percentage of affected persons who go on to develop schizophrenia is not known, but schizophrenia or paranoid psychosis is not the typical outcome.

369. The answer is a. *(Ebert, p 414.)* Vaginismus involves a spasm of the musculature of the outer one-third of the vagina and thereby interferes with sexual intercourse. Usually the spasm occurs in response to any attempted penetration, including vaginal examination. Some women with this disorder are able to become excited and reach orgasm through clitoral stimulation. The vaginal muscle spasm is not under voluntary control.

370. The answer is b. *(Ebert, pp 480–481.)* Avoidant personality disorder is characterized by pervasive and excessive hypersensitivity to negative evaluation, social inhibition, and feelings of inadequacy. Impairment can be severe due to social and occupational difficulties. Males and females are equally affected. The prevalence ranges from 0.5 to 1.5% in the general population. Among psychiatric outpatients, the prevalence is as high as 10%.

371. The answer is d. *(Ebert, pp 480–481.)* Avoidant personality disorder can be difficult to differentiate from social phobia. One differentiating factor is that in social phobia specific situations, rather than interpersonal contact, cause distress and are avoided.

372. The answer is d. *(Ebert, pp 419–420.)* In transvestite fetishism, patients, usually heterosexual males, experience recurrent and intense sexual arousal while they are cross-dressing. Masturbation with fantasies of sexual attractiveness while dressed as a woman usually accompanies the cross-dressing. Wearing an article of women's clothing or dressing as a woman while having intercourse can also be sexually exciting for these patients. The condition often begins in childhood or early adolescence. Males with this disorder consider themselves to be male, but some have gender dysphoria. For diagnostic purposes, the behavior must persist over a period of at least 6 months.

373. The answer is b. *(Ebert, pp 401–405.)* During periods of REM sleep, men experience penile erections defined as nocturnal penile tumescence (NPT). NPT studies can be helpful in differentiating patients with organic erectile problems from patients with psychogenic impotence. However, these findings are not absolute since many men have both organic and psychological causes for their impotence and nocturnal erections may be decreased or absent in depression. Since this patient has NPT, it is likely that his impotence stems from a psychogenic determinant, which may be reversible with treatment.

374. The answer is c. *(Ebert, pp 401–405.)* Polysomnography involves the recording of EEG activity during sleep, often combined with airflow measurements, ECG monitoring, eye movement monitoring, and electromyographic recording. Polysomnography does not include NPT studies.

375. The answer is b. *(Ebert, p 428.)* Chronic exposure to gastric juices through vomiting can cause severe erosion of the teeth and pathological pulp exposure in bulimic patients. Parotid gland enlargement is commonly observed in patients who binge and vomit. Esophageal tears, causing bloody emesis, can be a consequence of self-induced vomiting. The toxic effects of ipecac are cardiomyopathy and cardiac failure.

376–377. The answers are 376-b, 377-e. *(Ebert, pp 479–480.)* The essential feature of narcissistic personality disorder is a pervasive pattern of grandiosity, need for admiration, and lack of empathy that begins by early adulthood. Individuals with this disorder overestimate their abilities, inflate their accomplishments, and expect others to share the unrealistic opinion they have of themselves. They believe they are special and unique and attribute special qualities to those with whom they associate. When they do not receive the admiration they think they deserve, people with narcissistic personality react with anger and devaluation. The prevalence of the disorder is estimated at less than 1% of the general population, and 50 to 75% of those diagnosed with narcissistic personality are males. In contrast with their outward appearance, individuals with this disorder have a very vulnerable sense of self. Criticism leaves them feeling degraded and hollow. Narcissistic traits are common in adolescence, but most individuals do not progress to develop narcissistic personality disorder.

378. The answer is b. *(Ebert, pp 378–383.)* Factitious disorder is characterized by an intentional production of physical or psychological signs or symptoms with the intent to assume the sick role. Patients are usually unaware of their motivations, although they know their role in creating the illness. Factitious disorder is not synonymous with malingering. The external incentives that motivate malingering (avoiding work, avoiding unpleasant consequences, or obtaining compensation) are absent in factitious disorder. Multiple hospitalizations, invasive diagnostic procedures, and surgeries are common in the history of individuals with factitious disorder. The diagnosis may remain obscure for years, due to the covert nature of the disorder, the patient's habit of changing hospitals and doctors when suspicions are aroused, and the fact that, in some cases, genuine and feigned illnesses may coexist.

379. The answer is c. *(Ebert, p 584.)* Gender identity refers to a person's perception of the self as male or female. Biological, social, and psychological factors contribute to its development. By 2½ years of age, children can consistently identify themselves as male or female and recognize others as male or female. Sexual orientation refers to the individual's sexual response to males, females, or both. Gender dysphoria refers to the discontent with their biological sex experienced by individuals with gender identity disorder. Theory of the mind refers to children's awareness that others have cognitive processes and an internal mental status similar to their own and to their ability to represent the mental status of others in their own mind.

380–383. The answers are 380-f, 381-d, 382-b, 383-a. *(Ebert, pp 438–442, 444–446.)* Periodic limb movement disorder, once called nocturnal myoclonus, is characterized by very frequent, stereotyped limb movements, most often involving the legs. The movements are accompanied by brief arousal and disruption of sleep pattern, although the individual suffering from the disorder is only aware of being chronically tired during the day. Interviewing bed partners helps clarify the diagnosis. Circadian sleep disorders are characterized by insomnia and chronic sleepiness. They are due to a lack of synchrony between an individual's internal circadian sleep-wake cycles and the desired times of falling asleep and waking. The disorder can arise from an idiopathic variance in the periodic firing of the hypothalamic suprachiasmatic nucleus, which regulates the circadian cycles. The sleep cycles may be delayed, advanced, non-24-h, or irregular. Traveling through several time zones and work shifts requiring considerable changes in sleep patterns are also responsible for the disorder. Narcolepsy is a disorder of unknown origin characterized by an irresistible urge to fall asleep. Sleep attacks last from 10 to 20 min and may take place at very inopportune times. Patients may also experience cataplexy (sudden loss of muscle tone triggered by a strong emotion), hypnagogic hallucinations (hallucinations associated with falling asleep), and sleep paralysis (the individual is unable to move on arousal, a benign but frightening experience that represents an intrusion of REM-sleep phenomena into wakefulness). Primary hypersomnia is a chronic or recurrent disorder characterized by daytime sleepiness, excessive nighttime sleep, and need for daytime naps. Polysomnographic studies show an increase in slow-wave sleep. To make this diagnosis, other causes of daytime sleepiness without sleep deprivation must be ruled out.

384–387. The answers are 384-h, 385-e, 386-a, 387-d. *(Ebert, pp 416–420.)* Scatologia (becoming sexually aroused while making obscene phone calls) is categorized under paraphilias not otherwise specified, together with necrophilia (becoming aroused by dead bodies), zoophilia (sexual arousal triggered by animals), coprophilia (sexual arousal linked to touching or smelling feces), and many other forms of paraphilias. In exhibitionism, affected individuals become sexually aroused and sometimes masturbate while exposing their genitals to a stranger or while fantasizing about exposing themselves. There is no attempt to engage in a sexual activity with the stranger. Sometimes the individual is aroused by the stranger's surprise or shock; other times the exhibitionistic individual fantasizes that the observer will become sexually aroused. Frotteurism involves touching or rubbing against a nonconsenting person while fantasizing about having an exclusive relationship with that person. The behavior usually occurs in crowded places, such as on public transportation or busy sidewalks. In fetishism, the affected individual becomes sexually aroused and masturbates while holding, rubbing, or smelling a specific inanimate object. The fetish is required or strongly preferred for sexual excitement. This paraphilia usually starts by adolescence and, once established, tends to be chronic.

Substance-Related Disorders

Questions

DIRECTIONS: Each item below contains a question or incomplete statement followed by suggested responses. Select the **one best** response to each question.

Items 388–389

388. A 19-year-old man is brought to the emergency room by his distraught parents, who are worried about his vomiting and profuse diarrhea. On arrival, his pupils are dilated, his blood pressure is 175/105, and his muscles are twitching. His parents report that these symptoms started 2 h earlier. For the past few days he has been homebound due to a sprained ankle and, during this time, he has been increasingly anxious and restless. He has been yawning incessantly and has had a runny nose. Which of the following drugs is this man likely to be withdrawing from?

a. Heroin
b. Alcohol
c. PCP
d. Benzodiazepine
e. Cocaine

389. How long after cessation of use of this substance does its withdrawal syndrome usually peak?

a. 6 h
b. 15 h
c. 48 h
d. 3 days
e. 1 week

390. A 17-year-old boy is brought to the physician by his parents because they have noticed him becoming increasingly anxious, irritable, and hostile for the past 3 months. The boy adamantly states that there is nothing wrong with him. On physical exam, he is found to have acne, gynecomastia, and smaller than normal testicles and prostate. What substance has he most likely been abusing?

a. Methamphetamine
b. Heroin
c. Thyroxine
d. Testosterone
e. Estrogen

Items 391–392

391. A 50-year-old man is brought to the emergency department by ambulance. His respirations are shallow and infrequent, his pupils are constricted, and he is stuporous. He was noted to have suffered a grand mal seizure in the ambulance. Which of the following drugs is this man likely to have overdosed on?

a. Cocaine
b. LSD
c. Meperidine
d. PCP
e. MDMA (ecstasy)

392. After ensuring adequate ventilation for this patient, which of the following interventions should be next?

a. Intravenous naloxone
b. Intravenous phenobarbitol
c. Intravenous diazepam
d. Forced diuresis
e. Intramuscular haloperidol

393. A 22-year-old man arrives at an emergency room accompanied by several friends. He is agitated, confused, and apparently responding to frightening visual and auditory hallucinations. The patient is put in restraints after he tries to attack the emergency room physician. The patient's friends report that he had "dropped some acid" 6 or 7 h earlier. How much longer will intoxication with this substance last?

a. 1 to 6 h
b. 8 to 12 h
c. 14 to 18 h
d. 20 to 24 h
e. 26 to 30 h

Items 394–395

394. A college freshman, who has never consumed more than one occasional beer, is challenged to drink a large quantity of alcohol during his fraternity house's party. In a nontolerant person, signs of intoxication usually appear when the blood alcohol level reaches what range?

a. 20 to 30 mg/dL
b. 100 to 200 mg/dL
c. 300 mg/dL
d. 400 mg/dL
e. 500 mg/dL

395. The freshman goes home after drinking 6 cans of beer and falls asleep. What will be the effect of his drinking on his sleep?

a. There will be no effect
b. His REM sleep will be increased
c. His stage 4 sleep (deep sleep) will be increased
d. His sleep will be more fragmented
e. He will have shorter episodes of awakening

Items 396–397

396. A 35-year-old man stumbles into the emergency room. His pulse is 100/min, his blood pressure is 170/95 mmHg, and he is diaphoretic. He is tremulous and has difficulty relating a history. He does admit to insomnia the past two nights and sees spiders walking on the walls. He has been a drinker since age 19, but has not had a drink in 3 days. Which of the following is the most likely diagnosis?

a. Alcohol-induced psychotic disorder
b. Wernicke's psychosis
c. Alcohol withdrawal delirium
d. Alcohol intoxication
e. Alcohol idiosyncratic intoxication

397. Which of the following treatments should be initiated first?

a. Intramuscular haloperidol
b. Intramuscular chlorpromazine
c. Oral lithium
d. Oral chlordiazepoxide
e. Intravenous naloxone

Items 398–399

398. A 45-year-old housewife has been drinking in secret for several years. She started with one or two small glasses of Irish cream per night to help her sleep, but, with time, her nightly intake has increased to 4 to 5 hard liquor shots. Now she needs a few glasses of wine in the early afternoon to prevent shakiness and anxiety. During the past year, she could not take part in several important family events, including her son's high school graduation, because she was too ill or she did not want to risk missing her nightly drinking. She is ashamed of her secret and has tried to limit her alcohol intake but without success. Which of the following diagnoses is most likely?

a. Alcohol abuse
b. Alcohol addiction
c. Addictive personality disorder
d. Alcohol dependence
e. Alcohol-induced mood disorder

399. Which of the following statements about this diagnosis is correct?
a. Males and females have the same lifetime risk of developing this disorder
b. Race and religion do not affect its prevalence
c. Prevalence among Asians is considerably higher than among Caucasians
d. Native Americans have the lowest risk for this disorder among the United States' ethnic groups
e. Lifetime prevalence in women is 3 to 5%

400. Which nonopioid medication can be used to treat some of the symptoms of opioid withdrawal syndrome?
a. Chlordiazepoxide
b. Haloperidol
c. Methadone
d. Phenobarbital
e. Clonidine

401. A 24-year-old man is admitted for an appendectomy. The day after the surgery, he has a severe headache. Which one of his habits can best explain the headache?
a. He smokes one to two joints every other day
b. He drinks two to three beers once a week
c. He often eats at the local Chinese restaurant
d. He jogs three miles every day, rain or shine
e. He drinks five to six cups of coffee a day

Items 402–403

402. Three policemen, with difficulty, drag an agitated and very combative young man into an emergency room. Once there, he is restrained because he reacts with rage and tries to hit anyone who approaches him. When it is finally safe to approach him, the resident on call notices that the patient has very prominent vertical nystagmus. Shortly thereafter, the patient has a generalized seizure. Which of the following substances of abuse is the most likely to produce this presentation?
a. Amphetamine
b. PCP
c. Cocaine
d. Meperidine
e. LSD

403. Which of the following therapeutic interventions is most likely to be effective?

a. Naloxone administration
b. Urine alkalinization
c. Hemodialysis
d. Hyperbaric oxygen
e. Administration of a short-acting benzodiazepine

404. A factory worker is required to submit to random drug tests as part of the drug-free policy his employers have adopted. If he used cocaine 3 days before the test was administered, which assay is most likely to detect cocaine metabolites?

a. Blood
b. Hair
c. Saliva
d. Semen
e. Urine

405. Two policemen pull over the driver of a car, a 20-year-old man, for speeding. They immediately notice a strong smell of alcohol on his breath and administer a Breathalyzer test. According to the instrument, the man's blood alcohol level is 200 mg/dL, but he does not show any typical signs of intoxication. His gait is steady, his speech is clear, and he does not appear emotionally disinhibited. What is the most likely explanation for such presentation?

a. The Breathalyzer is defective
b. A value of 200 mg/dL is below the intoxication level
c. The man has developed a tolerance to the effects of alcohol
d. The man has alcohol dependence
e. The man has recently used cocaine, whose effects counteract the effects of alcohol intoxication

406. A woman swallows two amphetamines at a party and quickly becomes disinhibited and euphoric. Afterward, she slaps a casual acquaintance because she takes a benign comment as a major offense and starts raving about being persecuted. What mechanism is responsible for these behaviors?
a. Increased release of dopamine and norepinephrine in the synaptic cleft
b. Inhibition of catecholamine reuptake
c. Activation of NMDA receptors
d. Blockade of dopamine receptors
e. Sensitization of GABA receptors

407. A 25-year-old woman is dropped on the doorstep of a local emergency room by two men who immediately leave by car. She is agitated and anxious, and she keeps brushing her arms and legs "to get rid of the bugs." She clutches at her chest, moaning in pain. Her pupils are wide, and her BP is elevated. Which of the following substances is she most likely using?
a. Alcohol
b. Heroin
c. Alprazolam
d. LSD
e. Cocaine

408. A boy, both of whose biological parents are alcoholics, is adopted at birth by a couple who do not use alcohol. The adoptive parents ask the physician about their son's risk for alcoholism. Which of the following statements is true with regard to their adopted son's genetic risk for alcoholism compared to that of the general population?
a. The risk is 1.5 times higher
b. The risk is 3 to 4 times higher
c. The risk is 10 to 20 times higher
d. The risk is not elevated
e. The risk is elevated, but the exact figure is unknown

Items 409–410

409. A young woman becomes flushed and nauseated immediately after drinking half a glass of wine. This happens every time she consumes even a small quantity of alcohol. What is her race most likely to be?
a. Hispanic
b. Caucasian
c. Native American
d. African American
e. Asian

410. Which of the following mechanisms is the explanation for this reaction?
a. A problematic interaction between alcohol and a spice commonly used in this patient's country
b. A conditioned autonomic reaction due to strong cultural rules against alcohol
c. An inherited inactive acetaldehyde dehydrogenase enzyme
d. An inherited hypoactive variant of a P450 enzyme
e. An inherited inactive variant of alcohol dehydrogenase

411. Which of the following medications has been approved by the FDA for treatment of nicotine dependence?
a. Lithium
b. Clonazepam
c. Methylphenidate
d. Bupropion
e. Amitriptyline

412. Marijuana smoking impairs the operation of motor vehicles for how many hours after its use?
a. 20 to 30 min
b. 1 to 2 h
c. 4 to 6 h
d. 8 to 12 h
e. 24 h

Substance-Related Disorders 239

Items 413–414

413. A 16-year-old male with a long record of arrests for breaking and entering, assault and battery, and drug possession is found dead in his room with a plastic bag on his head. For several months he had been experiencing headaches, tremors, muscle weakness, unsteady gait, and tingling sensations in his hands and feet. These symptoms (and the manner the boy died) suggest that he was addicted to which substance?
a. PCP
b. Cocaine
c. Methamphetamine
d. An inhalant
e. Heroin

414. Which of the following statements about this substance is true?
a. Among eighth-graders, it is the most used substance after alcohol and nicotine
b. Accidental death is rare even among frequent users
c. Prevalence rates are higher among African Americans and Hispanics
d. Risk of addiction is very high, even after a single use
e. Medical complications are bothersome but not serious

415. A 27-year-old professional football player sees flashes of light and brightly colored triangles and circles on the white walls of his home. He also sees trailing images following moving objects and what seems to be a pattern in the air. He has had similar experiences in the past, mostly when he was ill or very tired. What past experience is more likely to be the cause of such perceptions?
a. He sniffed paint thinner twice at age 14
b. He used LSD four or five times at age 22
c. He smoked three to four joints every day from age 17 to 21
d. He drinks five to six cups of coffee a day
e. He used to binge on alcohol once a week during college years

416. The drug 3,4-methylenedioxymethamphetamine (MDMA), often known as ecstasy, causes which of the following effects?
a. A high lasting 5 to 7 days
b. Bruxism
c. Hypotension
d. An increased appetite
e. Suspiciousness and paranoia

Psychiatry

DIRECTIONS: Each group of questions below consists of lettered options followed by a set of numbered items. For each numbered item, select the **one** lettered option with which it is **most closely** associated. Each lettered option may be used once, more than once, or not at all.

Items 417–420

Match each definition with the correct term.

a. Tolerance
b. Potentiation
c. Withdrawal
d. Dependence
e. Addiction
f. Substance abuse

417. A maladaptive pattern of substance use that leads to clinically significant impairment or distress **(CHOOSE 1 TERM)**

418. Requirement of a larger dose of the drug to obtain the same effect **(CHOOSE 1 TERM)**

419. A physiologic state that follows cessation of or reduction in drug use **(CHOOSE 1 TERM)**

420. Interaction between two or more drugs resulting in a pharmacologic response greater than the sum of individual responses to each drug **(CHOOSE 1 TERM)**

Substance-Related Disorders

Answers

388. The answer is a. *(Ebert, p 247.)* Craving, anxiety, dysphoria, yawning, lacrimation, pupil dilatation, rhinorrhea, and restlessness are followed in more severe cases of withdrawal from short-acting drugs such as heroin or morphine by piloerection (cold turkey); twitching muscles and kicking movements of the lower extremities (kicking the habit); nausea; vomiting; diarrhea; low-grade fever; and increased blood pressure, pulse, and respiratory rate. Untreated, the syndrome resolves in 7 to 10 days. With longer-acting opiates, such as methadone, the onset of symptoms is delayed for 1 to 3 days after the last dose; peak symptoms do not occur until the third to eighth day, and symptoms may last for several weeks. Although very distressing, the opioid withdrawal syndrome is not life-threatening in healthy adults, but deaths have occurred in debilitated patients with other medical conditions.

389. The answer is c. *(Ebert, p 247.)* Withdrawal symptoms from short-acting drugs such as heroin or morphine can start within 8 to 12 h after the last dose and generally reach peak severity 48 h after the last dose.

390. The answer is d. *(Kaplan, 8/e, pp 454–455.)* Anabolic steroids include the natural male hormone testosterone and many synthetic analogues. They all have muscle-building (anabolic) and masculinizing (androgenic) effects. They are widely abused by individuals who want to increase their muscle mass and strength, to improve athletic performance, or to improve personal appearance. Irritability, aggressiveness, hypomania, and mania are common consequences of anabolic steroid abuse, especially in individuals taking large doses (1000 mg of testosterone equivalent per week or more). Psychotic symptoms have been described, but are much less common.

391. The answer is c. *(Ebert, p 247.)* Severe opiate intoxication is associated with respiratory depression, stupor or coma, and sometimes pulmonary edema. Less severe intoxication is associated with slurred speech, drowsiness, and impaired memory or attention. Early on, the pupils are constricted, but they dilate if the patient becomes anoxic due to the respiratory depression. Blood pressure is typically reduced. Meperidine intoxication in a chronic user is often complicated by delirium or seizures due to the accumulation of normeperidine, a toxic metabolite with cerebral irritant properties.

392. The answer is a. *(Kaplan, 8/e, p 442.)* Naloxone, an opiate antagonist, is used to reverse the effects of opiates. The first treatment intervention, however, is to ensure that the patient is adequately ventilated. Tracheopharyngeal secretions should be aspirated, and the patient should be mechanically ventilated until naloxone is administered and a positive effect on respiratory rate is noticed. The usual initial dose of naloxone is 0.8 mg slowly administered intravenously. If there is no response, the dose can be repeated every few minutes. In most cases of opiate intoxication, 4 to 5 mg of naloxone (total dose) are sufficient to reverse the CNS depression. Buprenorphine may require higher doses. Diazepam is used to treat alcohol withdrawal symptoms. Forced diuresis is used in the treatment of salicylates and acetaminophen overdoses, not opiate intoxication. Haloperidol, an antipsychotic medication, is not used for the acute treatment of opiate intoxication.

393. The answer is a. *(Ebert, p 248.)* Most cases of intoxication with a hallucinogen are over within 8 to 12 h, but prolonged drug-induced psychoses may occur, especially with phencyclidine (PCP), in which the psychosis may last several weeks.

394. The answer is a. *(Ebert, p 245.)* Behavioral changes, slowing of motor performance, and decrease in the ability to think clearly may appear with a blood alcohol level as low as 20 to 30 mg/dL. Most people show significant impairment of motor and mental performance when their alcohol levels reach 100 mg/dL. With blood alcohol concentration between 200 and 300 mg/dL, slurred speech is more intense and memory impairment, such as blackout and anterograde amnesia, becomes common. In a nontolerant person, a blood alcohol level over 400 mg/dL can produce respiratory failure, coma, and death. Due to tolerance, chronic heavy drinkers can present with fewer symptoms even with blood alcohol levels greater than 500 mg/dL.

Substance-Related Disorders *Answers* 243

395. The answer is d. *(Kaplan, 8/e, p 396.)* Alcohol consumption usually leads to an increased ease of falling asleep, but it has adverse effects on other parts of the sleep cycle. It decreases REM sleep, decreases stage 4 (deep) sleep, and increases sleep fragmentation. The notion of alcohol helping people sleep is a myth.

396. The answer is c. *(Ebert, pp 245–246.)* Alcohol withdrawal delirium (delirium tremens) is the most severe form of alcohol withdrawal. In this syndrome, coarse tremor of the hands, insomnia, anxiety, agitation, and autonomic hyperactivity (increased blood pressure and pulse, diaphoresis) are accompanied by severe agitation, confusion, and tactile or visual hallucinations. When alcohol use has been heavy and prolonged, withdrawal phenomena start within 8 h of cessation of drinking. Symptoms reach peak intensity between the second and the third day of abstinence and are usually markedly diminished by the fifth day. In a milder form, withdrawal symptoms may persist for weeks as part of a protracted syndrome. Wernicke's psychosis is an encephalopathy caused by severe thiamine deficiency, usually associated with prolonged and severe alcohol abuse. It is characterized by confusion, ataxia, and ophthalmoplegia. In alcohol hallucinosis, vivid auditory hallucinations start shortly after cessation or reduction of heavy alcohol use. Hallucinations may present with a clear sensorium and are accompanied by signs of autonomic instability less prominent than in alcohol withdrawal delirium.

397. The answer is d. *(Ebert, pp 245–246.)* Benzodiazepines are the preferred treatment for alcohol withdrawal delirium, with diazepam and chlordiazepoxide (Librium) the most commonly used. Elderly patients or patients with severe liver damage may better tolerate intermediate-acting benzodiazepines such as lorazepam and oxazepam. Thiamine (100 mg) and folic acid (1 mg) are routinely administered to prevent CNS damage secondary to vitamin deficiency. Thiamine should always be administered prior to glucose infusion, because glucose metabolism may rapidly deplete patients' thiamine reserves in cases of long-lasting poor nutrition. When the patient has a history of alcohol withdrawal seizures, magnesium sulfate should be administered.

398. The answer is d. *(Kaplan, 8/e, pp 397–399.)* A diagnosis of alcohol dependence requires the presence of compulsive drinking with ineffective attempts to stop or cut down; evidence of a severe impairment of occupational, social, and family life due to the great deal of time the patient spends procuring and consuming alcohol or recovering from its effects; persistent excessive drinking despite the problems alcohol causes; and physical symptoms and signs of withdrawal and tolerance.

399. The answer is e. *(Kaplan, 8/e, p 392.)* Three to five percent of the female population has a diagnosis of alcohol dependence. In males, the lifetime prevalence is estimated at 10%. Race, ethnicity, socioeconomic status, and religion greatly affect the prevalence of alcohol use and abuse. In the United States, Eskimos, Native Americans, and people of Irish descent have the highest rates of severe alcohol problems. Asians tend to have low rates of alcoholism due to a genetic variant of aldehyde dehydrogenase, which causes disulfiram-like symptoms after the ingestion of small quantities of alcohol.

400. The answer is e. *(Ebert, p 254.)* Clonidine, an α_2-adrenergic receptor agonist, is used to suppress some of the symptoms of mild opioid withdrawal. Clonidine is given orally, starting with doses of 0.1 to 0.3 mg three or four times a day. In outpatient settings, a daily dosage above 1 mg is not recommended due to the risk of severe hypotension. Clonidine is more effective on symptoms of autonomic instability, but is less effective than methadone in suppressing muscle aches, cravings, and insomnia. Clonidine is particularly useful in the detoxification of patients maintained on methadone.

401. The answer is e. *(Kaplan, 8/e, p 414.)* Postoperative headache due to caffeine withdrawal is a common occurrence, since patients are usually required to abstain from food and drink prior to surgery. Although the frequency and severity of withdrawal headaches increase with the daily dosage of caffeine consumed, caffeine withdrawal can occur even with a relatively low daily intake, such as 100 mg (the equivalent of one cup of brewed coffee) a day.

402. The answer is b. *(Ebert, p 256.)* Phencyclidine (PCP) intoxication is characterized by neurological, behavioral, cardiovascular, and autonomic manifestations. Intoxicated patients are often agitated, enraged, aggressive, and scared. Due to their exaggerated and distorted sensory input, they may have unpredictable and extreme reactions to environmental stimuli. Nystagmus and signs of neuronal hyperexcitability (from increased deep tendon reflexes to status epilepticus) and hypertension are typical findings.

403. The answer is e. *(Kaplan, 8/e, p 446.)* Benzodiazepines and dopamine receptor antagonists (antipsychotics) are the drugs of choice for controlling behavior pharmacologically. Hemodialysis is not effective due to the extremely large volume of distribution of PCP. Acidification and not alkalinization of urine has been used in an attempt to trap the ionized form of PCP in the urine, but the efficacy of this is controversial.

404. The answer is e. *(Ebert, p 250.)* All the listed body fluids except semen are used to detect cocaine use. Blood and saliva provide the best level of current usage, while urine assay detects use over the preceding several days. Hair analysis can reveal the drug over weeks or months, but has little clinical applicability.

405. The answer is c. *(Ebert, p 245.)* After prolonged use, most drugs of abuse (and some medications) produce adaptive changes in the brain that are manifested by a markedly diminished responsiveness to the effects of the substance that has been administered over time, a phenomenon called tolerance. Anyone who does not show signs of intoxication with an alcohol level of 150 mg/dL has developed a considerable tolerance.

406. The answer is a. *(Kaplan, 8/e, p 408.)* The main mechanism of action of amphetamines is the release of stored monoamines in the synaptic cleft. Cocaine inhibits the reuptake of the neurotransmitters released in the synapse. Benzodiazepines and barbiturates act by increasing the affinity of GABA type A receptors for their endogenous neurotransmitter, GABA. NMDA aspartate receptors are activated by PCP. Antipsychotic medications act by blocking dopamine receptors.

407. The answer is e. *(Ebert, p 246.)* Cocaine intoxication is characterized by euphoria but suspiciousness. Agitation, anxiety, and hyperactivity are also typical presenting symptoms. Signs of sympathetic stimulation, such as tachycardia, cardiac arrhythmias, hypertension, pupillary dilatations, perspiration, and chills are also present. Visual and tactile hallucinations, including hallucinations of bugs crawling on the skin, are present in cocaine-induced delirium. Among the most serious acute medical complications associated with the use of high doses of cocaine are coronary spasms, myocardial infarcts, intracranial hemorrhages, ischemic cerebral infarcts, and seizures.

408. The answer is b. *(Kaplan, 8/e, p 395.)* Many studies have shown that people with first-degree relatives affected with an alcohol-related disorder are 3 to 4 times more likely to have an alcohol-related disorder than people without such relatives. Adoptee studies have shown that the children of parents with alcohol-related disorders are at risk for an alcohol-related disorder even when brought up by families with parents without such disorders.

409–410. The answers are 409-e, 410-c. *(Kaplan, 8/e, p 396.)* Ten percent of Asian men and women lack the form of acetaldehyde dehydrogenase responsible for metabolizing low blood concentrations of acetaldehyde (they are homozygous for an inactive form of the enzyme). Approximately 40% of Asian men and women are heterozygous for this specific enzyme variation. Due to the rapid accumulation of acetaldehyde, homozygous individuals develop facial flushing, nausea, and vomiting after ingestion of small quantities of alcohol. Heterozygous individuals can tolerate some alcohol, but are more sensitive to its effects. This enzyme variation is found only in Asian people.

411. The answer is d. *(Kaplan, 8/e, p 435.)* A variety of psychopharmacologic agents, including clonidine, antidepressants, and buspirone, have been used with some success in the treatment of nicotine dependence. Bupropion (Zyban) was approved by the FDA in 1996 for this use.

412. The answer is d. *(Kaplan, 8/e, p 418.)* Marijuana has been clearly demonstrated to decrease judgment, impair ability to estimate time and distance, and impair motor function. As with alcohol, these effects make accidents one of the major dangers of smoking marijuana. These two substances may also potentiate each other. Up to 17% of drivers in fatal accidents have tested positive for cannabinoids. Driving ability is significantly affected for 8 to 12 h after smoking, and the ability of experienced pilots to fly is significantly decreased for 24 h.

413. The answer is d. *(Kaplan, 8/e, p 432.)* Inhalant abuse is associated with very serious medical problems. Hearing loss, peripheral neuritis, paresthesias, cerebellar signs, and motor impairment are common neurological manifestations. Muscle weakness due to rhabdomyolysis, irreversible hepatic and renal damage, cardiovascular symptoms, and gastrointestinal symptoms such as vomiting and hematemesis are also common in chronic severe abuse.

414. The answer is a. *(Kaplan, 8/e, p 430.)* Many adolescents experiment with inhalants. Among eighth-graders, inhalants are second only to nicotine and alcohol as a drug of abuse, but only a few become chronic users and maintain the habit into adulthood. Death by asphyxiation, aspiration, respiratory depression, arrhythmias, and accidents is a significant risk among chronic users.

415. The answer is b. *(Kaplan, 8/e, p 428.)* Hallucinogen-induced visual disturbances may persist for years after cessation of drug use. Sporadic visual symptoms are called flashbacks, while more lingering hallucinations are considered to be a hallucinogenic persistent perception disorder. These disorders are not dose-dependent and may develop after a single use. Perceptual symptoms include geometric hallucinations, flashes of color, and afterimages. Patients often complain about the persistence of trailing images while an object moves through the visual field. The entire visual field may be described as grainy or reticulated, and patients at times complain that they "can see the air." Patients' reality testing is intact and they know that their perceptions are not real. Symptoms are triggered by stimulants, including caffeine and decongestants, marijuana, fatigue, and infections. Most people recover completely in 5 years, but for others symptoms may be irreversible.

416. The answer is b. *(Kaplan, 8/e, p 410.)* MDMA (ecstasy) was tried in the 1970s as an adjunct to psychotherapy and later became popular as a recreational drug. After ingestion there is an initial phase of disorientation, followed by a "rush" that includes increased blood pressure and pulse rate as well as sweating. Users experience euphoria, increased self-confidence, and peaceful feelings of empathy and closeness to other people. Effects usually last 4 to 6 h. MDMA decreases appetite. It has been associated with bruxism (grinding of the teeth), shortness of breath, cardiac arrhythmia, and death.

417–420. The answers are 417-f, 418-a, 419-c, 420-b. *(Kaplan, 8/e, pp 375–378.)* These terms are commonly confused or used ambiguously. Substance abuse describes a maladaptive behavioral pattern characterized by recurrent use in spite of academic, social, or work problems; use in situations in which changes in mental status may be dangerous (driving); and recurrent substance-related legal problems. Tolerance refers to the pharmacological adaptation due to which a larger dose of a drug becomes necessary over time to achieve the same effect. Dependence is a condition in which withdrawal symptoms occur if the drug is stopped, usually leading to further drug use despite adverse consequences. With respect to drugs of abuse, tolerance and dependence often coexist. Withdrawal refers to a substance-specific syndrome that occurs after the cessation of the substance whose use has been heavy and prolonged. An example of the use of potentiation for clinical benefit is the coadministration of a benzodiazepine and an antipsychotic to an agitated psychotic patient. Both medications can be used at lower doses when used together than either could if used alone.

Psychopharmacology and Other Somatic Therapies

Questions

DIRECTIONS: Each item below contains a question or incomplete statement followed by suggested responses. Select the **one best** response to each question.

Items 421–422

421. A young man with a psychotic disorder is started on a neuroleptic medication. Two days after the beginning of the treatment, he cannot stop pacing and is unable to sit still. He reports that he feels jittery and complains that his legs are moving on their own. Which of the following statements is true with regard to these symptoms?

a. They are a rare neuroleptic side effect
b. They are an indication that the medication is not working and needs to be increased
c. They most often occur shortly after the initiation of neuroleptics
d. They are well tolerated by most patients
e. They are associated with an increased risk of neuroleptic malignant syndrome

422. Which of the following medications is most likely to prove helpful with the symptoms of this patient?

a. Beta blocker
b. Phenytoin
c. Amantadine
d. Benztropine
e. Higher-potency neuroleptic

423. A 25-year-old man with major depression discusses the potential benefits and side effects of various antidepressants with his psychiatrist. He clearly indicates that he does not want a medication that could decrease his libido or interfere with his ability to obtain and maintain an erection. Which of the listed antidepressants would be appropriate for this patient?

a. Bupropion
b. Clomipramine
c. Amitriptyline
d. Sertraline
e. Paroxetine

424. Which of the following drugs is a tricyclic antidepressant?

a. Fluoxetine
b. Nortriptyline
c. Phenelzine
d. Tranylcypromine
e. Clonazepam

425. A 12-year-old boy is very distraught because every time he thinks or hears the word *God* or passes in front of a church, swear words pop into his mind against his will. He also feels compelled to repeat the end of every sentence twice and to count to 20 before answering any question. If he is interrupted, he has to start from the beginning. Which of the following medications has been proven effective with this disorder?

a. Alprazolam
b. Clomipramine
c. Propranolol
d. Phenobarbital
e. Lithium

426. A 7-year-old boy is brought to the physician with a 1-year history of making careless mistakes and not listening in class and at home. He is easily distracted and forgetful and loses his schoolbooks often. He is noted to be fidgety, talking excessively and interrupting others. Which of the following medications is most likely to be helpful with this boy's symptoms?

a. Haloperidol
b. Alprazolam
c. Lithium
d. Methylphenidate
e. Paroxetine

427. A 19-year-old man is diagnosed with paranoid schizophrenia. He has command auditory hallucinations and persecutory delusions, but is also apathetic and withdrawn, with a flat affect. Which of the following medications is most likely to treat both the positive and the negative symptoms of this patient?
a. Chlorpromazine
b. Fluphenazine
c. Olanzapine
d. Quetiapine
e. Trifluoperazine

428. Which of the following statements best describes the half-life of a drug during steady-state conditions?
a. The expiration date of the drug
b. How long it takes to absorb the drug following ingestion
c. How long the drug will remain at least 50% active
d. How long it will take to metabolize one-half the drug
e. How long it will take before the medication has half the desired effect

429. Which of the following antidepressants is relatively contraindicated in young men secondary to its side effect of priapism?
a. Amitriptyline
b. Imipramine
c. Sertraline
d. Venlafaxine
e. Trazodone

430. In TCA overdose, which of the following dose levels will likely prove fatal if ingested? (Pick the lowest dose range likely to be fatal in over 50% of patients.)
a. 250 to 500 mg
b. 500 to 750 mg
c. 1 to 2 g
d. 2 to 3 g
e. 4 to 6 g

252 Psychiatry

431. A 78-year-old man with Parkinson's disease and a past history of recurrent depression has been increasingly sad, tearful, and withdrawn for several weeks. He has stopped eating to atone for past sins and hears the voice of the devil telling him that he will be damned for all eternity because he has failed his family and God. He is hospitalized after an unsuccessful attempt to kill himself by hanging. Since in the past the patient has not had a good response to antidepressants, and given the seriousness of his status, ECT is recommended. Which of the following statements about ECT is true?

a. ECT is associated with a relatively high mortality in older people
b. ECT is very effective in severe, psychotic depression
c. ECT is not as effective as antidepressants
d. ECT is contraindicated in patients with Parkinson's disease
e. ECT is not effective in psychiatric disorders other than depression

432. A 30-year-old male has taken sertraline 100 mg/d for the past 8 months as treatment for dysthymic disorder. Decreased libido and delayed orgasm have been a problem since the beginning of the treatment, but for a while the patient tolerated these side effects because, thanks to the medication, he has felt happier, more confident, and more energetic. He now presents to his psychiatrist's office reporting that, since he is getting married, these sexual side effects represent a more serious problem. He does not want to change antidepressants because, aside from the sexual problems, he is pleased with its effects. Which of the following medications could be helpful in these circumstances?

a. Clonazepam
b. Amitriptyline
c. Propranolol
d. Fluoxetine
e. Cyproheptadine

433. Which of the following statements best describes a double-blind, placebo-controlled crossover treatment study?

a. The subject does not know whether he or she is getting drug or placebo during the study and is not told after completion of the study
b. The researcher does not know if the subject is getting drug or placebo and is not told after completion of the study
c. The subject is not told what he or she is taking and is switched from drug to placebo in mid-study
d. Neither the patient nor the researcher knows whether drug or placebo is being used, and a switch is made in mid-study
e. The researcher is not told whether placebo or drug is being used, and a switch is made at mid-study

Items 434–435

434. A 48-year-old woman with a past history of recurrent psychotic depression is admitted to a locked ward during a relapse. On the day of admission, she is placed on nortriptyline 50 mg and risperidone 2 mg at bedtime. Ten days later, the patient reports with great concern that her nipples are leaking. Which class of medications is known to cause this condition?

a. Benzodiazepines
b. Neuroleptics
c. Serotonin reuptake inhibitors
d. Antiseizure medications with mood-stabilizing properties
e. Beta blockers

435. What mechanism is responsible for the condition?

a. Excessive release of monoamines in the synaptic cleft
b. Blockage of serotonin reuptake
c. Activation of NMDA receptors
d. Dopamine receptor blockade
e. Sensitization of GABA receptors to the agonistic effects of endogenous GABA

254 Psychiatry

436. A 56-year-old woman is brought to the emergency department by her relatives after she was found tremulous, ataxic, and somnolent. Her lithium level is 1.8 meq/L. There was no change in her lithium dosage recently, and she is not dehydrated. Her family states that during the past week the patient has been taking several daily doses of an over-the-counter medication. Which medication did the patient take in addition to her lithium?

a. Acetylsalicylate
b. Acetaminophen
c. Ibuprofen
d. Diphenhydramine
e. Pseudoephedrine

437. Which of the following benzodiazepines has the shortest half-life?

a. Alprazolam
b. Lorazepam
c. Flurazepam
d. Diazepam
e. Triazolam

438. Which of the following antipsychotic medications is the most potent?

a. Chlorpromazine
b. Thiothixene
c. Trifluoperazine
d. Haloperidol
e. Thioridazine

439. A 35-year-old woman with bipolar disorder has been stable on lithium for 2 years. For the past 3 months, she has been easily fatigued, more sensitive to cold, and excessively sleepy. Her hair is dry and brittle, and her face is puffy. Which of the following lab results will most likely be found?

a. Elevated TSH
b. Elevated liver function tests
c. Leukopenia
d. Blunted cortisol response to ACTH
e. Hypocholesterolemia

440. A 25-year-old woman with bipolar disorder develops a high fever with chills, bleeding gums, extreme fatigue, and pallor 3 weeks after starting on carbamazepine. Which of the following is she experiencing?
a. Stevens-Johnson syndrome
b. Acute aplastic anemia
c. Serotonin syndrome
d. Neuroleptic malignant syndrome
e. Malignant hyperthermia

441. A 26-year-old man with paranoid schizophrenia remains severely psychotic after several trials of typical and atypical neuroleptics. He has received haloperidol, perphenazine, molindone, risperidone, and olanzapine at optimal therapeutic dosages, but his thought processes remain disorganized. He continues to believe that malevolent entities poison his water and his food, and he has assaulted at least one person in response to command auditory hallucinations. Which of the following medications should be tried next?
a. Loxapine
b. Thioridazine
c. Quetiapine
d. Clozapine
e. Fluphenazine

442. A 22-year-old man is being treated with fluoxetine for major depression. Hoping to become less depressed more quickly, he also begins taking a relative's phenelzine, a monoamine oxidase inhibitor (MAOI). Two days later he is brought to the emergency department after becoming confused. He also complains of visual hallucinations and myoclonic jerks. On physical examination, he is flushed and diaphoretic. His temperature is 39.5°C (103°F). Which of the following is the most likely diagnosis?
a. Meningitis
b. Overdose of fluoxetine
c. Neuroleptic malignant syndrome
d. Serotonin syndrome
e. Extrapyramidal side effect

443. A 42-year-old man is diagnosed with a psychotic depression and is started on imipramine and perphenazine. When he develops a dystonia, he is begun on benztropine 2 mg/d. One week later, his wife reports that the patient has become unusually forgetful and seems disoriented at night. On physical examination, the man appears slightly flushed, his skin and palms are dry, and he is tachycardic. He is oriented to name and place only. He showed none of these symptoms during his last appointment. Which of the following diagnoses is most likely?

a. Anticholinergic syndrome
b. Neuroleptic malignant syndrome
c. Extrapyramidal side effect
d. Akathisia
e. Dementia

444. A 43-year-old high school teacher becomes despondent, tearful, and withdrawn 2 weeks after starting a medication for her arthritis prescribed by her family doctor. Which of the following medications is likely to cause these symptoms?

a. Ibuprofen
b. Cortisone
c. Acetaminophen
d. Acetylsalicylate
e. Imipramine

445. A 56-year-old woman who was diagnosed with paranoid schizophrenia in her early twenties has received daily doses of various typical neuroleptics for many years. For the past 2 years, she has had symptoms of tardive dyskinesia. Discontinuation of the neuroleptic is not possible because she becomes aggressive and violent in response to command hallucinations when she is not medicated. Which of the following actions should be taken next?

a. Start the patient on benztropine
b. Start the patient on amantadine
c. Start the patient on propranolol
d. Start the patient on diphenhydramine
e. Switch the patient to clozapine

446. Which of the following is the best indicator of the severity of a tricyclic overdose?
a. Pupillary reactivity
b. Fluctuation of body temperature
c. QRS prolongation
d. Liver transaminase level
e. Respiratory rate

447. A 32-year-old man with treatment-resistant schizophrenia is started on clozapine. He is informed that his blood will need to be drawn weekly. Which of the following tests should be ordered when the blood is drawn?
a. Sodium
b. White blood cell count
c. Creatinine
d. Platelets
e. Red blood cell count

448. The mechanism of action of antipsychotic drugs is believed to involve blockade at receptor sites for which of the following compounds?
a. Histamine
b. Dopamine
c. Acetylcholine
d. Epinephrine
e. γ-aminobutyric acid

449. A 32-year-old woman with bipolar disorder gives birth to a full-term female infant with spina bifida. Which of the following medications is most likely responsible for this defect if taken in the first trimester?
a. Sertraline
b. Perphenazine
c. Clonazepam
d. Lithium
e. Valproate

450. A 45-year-old homeless man with paranoid schizophrenia has been repeatedly noncompliant with his oral antipsychotic medications. During his last hospitalization, he agreed to switch from his oral preparation of fluphenazine to an injectable, long-acting form. He received his first injection of the medication without incident. When should the next injection be scheduled?

a. 24 h
b. 3 days
c. 2 weeks
d. 2 months
e. 4 months

451. A 72-year-old man develops acute urinary retention and blurred vision after taking an antidepressant for 3 days. Which medication is most likely to cause such side effects?

a. Venlafaxine
b. Paroxetine
c. Bupropion
d. Nefazodone
e. Amitriptyline

452. A 28-year-old man with bipolar disorder was started on fluoxetine 20 mg/d after he became depressed. He had previously been maintained on carbamazepine 100 mg/d, which was continued. One month after he began the fluoxetine, blood levels of carbamazepine returned supratherapeutic. The patient's carbamazepine level had previously always been therapeutic, and he reported taking the medication as he always had. Which of the following possibilities is most likely the explanation for the finding of a supratherapeutic carbamazepine level?

a. The patient is not accurately taking the medication
b. Fluoxetine is slowing the metabolism of carbamazepine
c. The fluoxetine is interacting with the CYP 3A4 enzyme
d. The carbamazepine is being excreted more slowly
e. The carbamazepine is inhibiting the excretion of the fluoxetine

453. A 9-year-old girl has significant social difficulties due to her unusual behaviors. Her grunts, her motor tics, and coprolalia are a constant cause of embarrassment and shame. What medication can relieve her symptoms?

a. Methylphenidate
b. Clomipramine
c. Sertraline
d. Trazodone
e. Haloperidol

454. An 8-year-old boy has been constantly clearing his throat and blinking his eyes for the past 3 weeks. He has had these symptoms intermittently for several years and has never been completely free of them for more than a day or two. Which of the following medications should be considered?

a. Alprazolam
b. Methylphenidate
c. Haloperidol
d. Amitriptyline
e. Lithium

455. During a 2-month period, a 72-year-old woman who has senile dementia becomes increasingly withdrawn, shows little interest in food, has trouble sleeping, and appears to become more severely demented. Her medical status is unchanged. Which of the following courses of treatment would be the most reasonable?

a. Diphenhydramine at bedtime to improve sleep
b. Diazepam three times daily
c. Imipramine at night
d. Perphenazine at bedtime
e. Sertraline in the morning

Items 456–457

456. A 34-year-old woman with a history of alcohol abuse has her first relapse after 2 years of sobriety. Fearing that she may not be able to stay away from alcohol, she asks her primary care physician to prescribe disulfiram. The following week she arrives at the emergency room with facial flushing, hypotension, tachycardia, nausea, and vomiting. She denies any recent ingestion of alcohol. What could have caused her symptoms?

a. Aged cheese
b. Cough syrup
c. An overripe mango
d. Two 30-mg tablets of pseudoephedrine
e. A bar of chocolate

457. The effect of disulfiram depends on which of the following mechanisms?

a. Monoamine oxidase inhibition
b. Lactate dehydrogenase inhibition
c. Dopamine receptor blockade
d. α_2 receptor antagonism
e. Acetaldehyde dehydrogenase inhibition

458. A 24-year-old man comes to see his physician after he is involved in a serious car crash because he fell asleep while driving. For several years, he has had severe daytime sleepiness, episodes of falling asleep without warning, and hypnagogic hallucinations. Which of the following medications should this patient be given?

a. Melatonin
b. Clonazepam
c. Methylphenidate
d. Thyroxine
e. Bromocriptine

459. For several weeks, a 72-year-old retired physician with Parkinson's disease and mild dementia has been talking about "those horrible people that come to bother me every night." He is convinced that someone is plotting against him, and he has nailed his window shut for fear of intruders. More recently, he has started showing signs of thought disorder, mostly in the evening and at night. Which of the following antipsychotic medications is least likely to worsen the patient's Parkinsonism?

a. Haloperidol
b. Perphenazine
c. Fluphenazine
d. Clozapine
e. Chlorpromazine

460. A 35-year-old man is diagnosed with a major depression and started on sertraline 25 mg/d. After 1 week the sertraline is increased to 50 mg/d. The patient remains depressed and does not respond to the sertraline. After 2 weeks on the sertraline with no response (first at 25 mg and then at 50 mg), what is the most appropriate next step?

a. Stop the sertraline and begin fluoxetine
b. Add lithium to the sertraline
c. Increase the sertraline
d. Add methylphenidate to the sertraline
e. Stop the sertraline and begin desipramine

Items 461–462

461. A 29-year-old woman with a previous diagnosis of bipolar disorder is hospitalized during an acute manic episode. She is elated, sexually provocative, and speaks very fast, jumping from one subject to the other. She tells the nurses that she has been chosen by God to be "the second virgin Mary." BUN, creatinine, electrolytes, TSH, and an ECG are within normal limits. What other test is necessary before starting the patient on lithium?

a. Pregnancy test
b. Total bilirubin
c. EEG
d. Iron-binding capacity
e. Chest x-ray

462. After appropriate tests are obtained, lithium treatment is started. Within what time interval does this medication come to steady state with regular administration?

a. Less than 24 h
b. 1 to 4 days
c. 5 to 8 days
d. 2 to 3 weeks
e. 1 to 2 months

463. A 25-year-old kindergarten teacher has been asked to run a group for parents once a month. Although pleased with this opportunity, she experiences severe anticipatory anxiety. At the beginning of the first meeting, her heart starts pounding, her mouth is dry, and she is so anxious that she has to ask a colleague to take her place. She consults a psychiatrist, who recommends propranolol, to be taken before the feared meetings. In which of the following medical conditions would this medication be contraindicated for this patient?

a. Obesity
b. Asthma
c. Alcohol abuse
d. Hypertension
e. Breast cancer

464. Which of the following hormones is used in the adjuvant treatment of depression?

a. Progesterone
b. Cortisol
c. ACTH
d. Levothyroxine
e. Prolactin

465. A 32-year-old woman is prescribed nortriptyline for her first episode of major depression. The initial dose is 25 mg at bedtime, gradually increased over the next week to 50 mg at bedtime. Two days after the dosage increase, the woman develops urinary retention, blurred vision, and severe constipation. Her blood level is 280 ng/mL (recommended therapeutic window is 50 to 150 ng/mL) 12 h after the last dose. What can explain this toxic blood level?

a. The patient smokes 15 cigarettes a day
b. The patient takes carbamazepine 200 mg three times a day to treat trigeminal neuralgia
c. The prescribed dose is excessively high
d. The patient has taken 800 mg of ibuprofen every day for the past week for headaches
e. The patient is a poor metabolizer

466. A patient with refractory schizophrenia has been almost free of active psychotic symptoms and has been functioning considerably better since he was placed on clozapine 500 mg/d, but he has experienced two episodes of grand mal seizure. What is the best course of action to take next?

a. Discontinue the clozapine and begin another antipsychotic
b. Decrease the clozapine
c. Stop the clozapine and start valproic acid
d. Add tegretol to the clozapine
e. Temporarily stop the clozapine and start phenobarbitol

467. A patient reports that she has become depressed with the onset of winter every year for the past 6 years. Which of the following treatments is most likely to be helpful with this patient?

a. Phototherapy
b. Biofeedback
c. Electroconvulsive therapy
d. Benzodiazepines
e. Steroid medication

468. A 19-year-old girl is taken hostage with other bystanders during an armed robbery. She is freed by police intervention after 10 h of captivity, but only after she has witnessed the shooting death of two of her captors. Months after this event, she has flashbacks and frightening nightmares. She startles at every noise and experiences acute anxiety whenever she is reminded of the robbery. Which of the following medications may help decrease this patient's hyperarousal?

a. Clonidine
b. Methylphenidate
c. Bupropion
d. Valproate
e. Thioridazine

469. A 72-year-old man with a long history of recurrent psychotic depression is hospitalized during a relapse. He has prostatic hypertrophy, coronary heart disease, and recurrent orthostatic hypotension. Which is the most appropriate antipsychotic medication for this patient?

a. Chlorpromazine
b. Clozapine
c. Thioridazine
d. Haloperidol
e. Olanzapine

470. A 47-year-old businessman who has taken paroxetine 40 mg/d for 6 months for depression leaves for a 2-week business trip overseas and forgets his medication at home. Since his depression has been in full remission for at least 3 months, he decides to stop the treatment without talking with his psychiatrist. Two days later, he becomes very irritable, tearful, dizzy, and nauseated. He shivers and feels like he has a bad cold. What is the cause of such symptoms?

a. Relapse of his major depression
b. Serotonin syndrome
c. SSRI discontinuation syndrome
d. Manic episode
e. Jet lag

471. The benzodiazepines' action depends on their interaction with which of the following receptors?

a. GABA
b. Serotonin
c. NMDA-glutamate
d. Dopamine
e. Acetylcholine

Items 472–473

472. A 42-year-old woman with atypical depression who has responded well to an MAOI presents to an emergency room with severe headache. Her blood pressure is 180/110. She states that she has been carefully avoiding high-tyramine foods as she was told, but admits that a friend gave her two tablets of a cold medication shortly before her symptoms started. What over-the-counter medication is contraindicated with MAOI treatment?

a. Pseudoephedrine
b. Acetaminophen
c. Diphenhydramine
d. Ibuprofen
e. Guaifenesin

473. If the woman's symptoms were due to a dietary indiscretion, what food would be the most probable cause of her symptoms?

a. Two slices of pepperoni pizza
b. A bagel with cream cheese
c. Three ounces of grilled fresh meat
d. Three fresh apples
e. A serving of fresh grilled cod

474. A 28-year-old woman is embarrassed by her peculiar tendency to collapse on the floor whenever she feels strong emotion. Since this disorder is caused by REM sleep intrusion during daytime, a neurologist prescribes a medication that reduces and delays REM sleep. Which of the following medications is likely to have been chosen?

a. Clonazepam
b. Methylphenidate
c. Pimozide
d. Desipramine
e. L-dopa

Items 475–476

475. A mentally retarded male adolescent who has been increasingly aggressive and agitated receives several consecutive IM doses of haloperidol, totaling 30 mg in 24 h, as a chemical restraint. The next day, he is rigid, confused, and unresponsive. His blood pressure is 150/95, his pulse is 110/min, and his temperature is 102°F. His white blood cell (WBC) count is 25,000, and CPK level is 1,200 μ/L. What is the most likely diagnosis?

a. Acute dystonic reaction
b. Neuroleptic-induced Parkinson's disease
c. Malignant hyperthermia
d. Neuroleptic malignant syndrome
e. Catatonia

476. What medication can be effective in treating this condition?

a. Bromocriptine
b. Carbamazepine
c. Chlorpromazine
d. Lithium
e. Propranolol

477. A 7-year-old boy who wets the bed at least three times a week and has not responded to appropriate behavioral interventions is diagnosed with ADHD. What medication is indicated to treat both disorders?

a. Bupropion
b. Dextroamphetamine
c. Clonidine
d. Risperidone
e. Imipramine

478. A 72-year-old retired college professor's memory and cognitive functions have slowly but progressively deteriorated for over 2 years. His wife asks his doctor for a medication that can slow her husband's decline. Which class of medications may slow the development of the symptoms of dementia?
a. Serotonin reuptake inhibitors
b. TCAs
c. Atypical neuroleptics
d. Cholinesterase inhibitors
e. Beta blockers

479. Which of the following serum level ranges is the target for lithium use in acute mania?
a. 0.5 to 1.0 meq/L
b. 1.0 to 1.5 meq/L
c. 1.5 to 2.0 meq/L
d. 2.0 to 2.5 meq/L
e. 2.5 to 3.0 meq/L

480. Which of the following cardiovascular effects can be most problematic secondary to TCA use?
a. Decreased myocardial contractility
b. Slowing of cardiac conduction
c. Increased risk for cardiac ischemia
d. Toxic myocardiopathy
e. Thickening of mitral valve cusps

DIRECTIONS: Each group of questions below consists of lettered options followed by a set of numbered items. For each numbered item, select the **one** lettered option with which it is **most closely** associated. Each option can be chosen once, more than once, or not at all.

Items 481–484

For each patient's symptoms, select the most likely diagnosis.
a. Parkinsonian tremor
b. Akathisia
c. Neuroleptic malignant syndrome
d. Dystonia
e. Anticholinergic syndrome
f. Seizure activity
g. Rabbit syndrome
h. Lithium-induced tremor
i. Akinesia

481. A 35-year-old painter with bipolar disorder is very frustrated by a fine tremor of her hands that worsens when she works and makes her smudge her paintings. **(SELECT 1 DIAGNOSIS)**

482. An 18-year-old male is admitted to a locked psychiatric unit after he assaulted his father. He is convinced that his family members have been substituted with malevolent aliens and hears several voices that comment on his actions and call him demeaning names. Two days after initiating treatment, he develops a painful spasm of the neck muscles and his eyes are forced in an upward gaze. **(SELECT 1 DIAGNOSIS)**

483. A 55-year-old man diagnosed with schizophrenia in adolescence has been successfully treated with medications for many years. He has a coarse, pill-rolling tremor that worsens at rest and improves during voluntary movements. **(SELECT 1 DIAGNOSIS)**

484. A 45-year-old woman with schizoaffective disorder has received neuroleptic medications, antidepressants, and mood stabilizers for at least 20 years. She presents with very rapid chewing movements. Other facial muscles, her trunk, and extremities are not affected, and her tongue does not dart in and out of her mouth when she is asked to protrude it. **(SELECT 1 DIAGNOSIS)**

Psychopharmacology and Other Somatic Therapies

Answers

421. The answer is c. *(Stoudemire, 3/e, pp 644–645.)* Akathisia is characterized by a subjective feeling of restlessness and an inability to stay still. This disorder manifests itself with pacing, shifting of position, and constant leg movements. Akathisia is a very common side effect of neuroleptic treatment, with a prevalence estimated between 20 and 75%. It usually arises during the first few days of treatment and is more frequent in individuals with a recent onset of psychosis. High-potency typical neuroleptics are more likely to cause akathisia than low-potency typical antipsychotic medications. Although atypical neuroleptic medications have a considerably lower prevalence of akathisia, occasionally they do have this side effect. Akathisia can be very distressing and can be a cause of treatment noncompliance. It can also be misdiagnosed for a worsening of the psychotic illness. In these cases, it gets worse when the neuroleptic that precipitated the syndrome is increased.

422. The answer is a. *(Stoudemire, 3/e, pp 644–645.)* Beta blockers, especially propranolol, are the treatment of choice in akathisia. More selective beta blockers such as atenolol and metoprolol have the advantage of not triggering bronchospasm in susceptible patients, but they appear to be less effective than propranolol.

423. The answer is a. *(Kaplan, 8/e, pp 1000–1004.)* Tricyclic antidepressants such as clomipramine and amitriptyline and SSRIs such as paroxetine and sertraline, as well as MAOIs, can cause erectile dysfunction, delayed ejaculation, anorgasmia, and decreased libido. Bupropion, mirtazapine, trazodone, and nefazodone, in contrast, do not affect sexual functions in a negative way. Trazodone and nefazodone, however, have been implicated in cases of priapism and should not therefore be used as first-line medications in male patients.

424. The answer is b. *(Kaplan, 8/e, p 1107.)* The tricyclic drugs include imipramine, desipramine, amitriptyline, and nortriptyline. They are effective in the treatment of depression; several anxiety disorders including panic disorder, generalized anxiety disorder, and separation anxiety; enuresis; and ADHD. Clomipramine, a TCA with serotonin reuptake–inhibiting properties, is effective in the treatment of obsessive-compulsive disorder. Tricyclic antidepressants have different side effect profiles, with each blocking cholinergic, adrenergic, and histaminic receptors to different degrees. For example, desipramine has less anticholinergic activity than imipramine, and nortriptyline is less likely to cause orthostatic hypotension than amitriptyline. Phenelzine and tranylcypromine are both MAO inhibitors, and clonazepam is a long-acting benzodiazepine.

425. The answer is b. *(Kaplan, 8/e, pp 1105–1106.)* Clomipramine is a tricyclic antidepressant effective in the treatment of obsessive-compulsive disorder in both children and adults. Its efficacy is thought to be related to its effects on inhibition of serotonin reuptake. SSRIs are also effective medications for the treatment of OCD.

426. The answer is d. *(Kaplan, 8/e, p 1197.)* This young boy suffers from Attention-Deficit/Hyperactivity Disorder (ADHD). The treatment of choice in ADHD is CNS stimulants, primarily detroamphetamine, methylphenidate, and pemoline.

427. The answer is c. *(Ebert, pp 272–274.)* Olanzepine and clozapine are the only antipsychotic medications that ameliorate both negative and positive symptoms in schizophrenic patients. Both are associated with fewer relapses and an improvement in quality of life, but olanzapine has a more benign side effect profile than clozapine.

428. The answer is d. *(Kaplan, 8/e, p 934.)* The elimination half-life of a drug, usually referred to as simply the half-life, refers to how long it will take the body to metabolize one-half of the drug. A steady state exists when, after a period of continued dosing, the quantity of medication entering the body equals the amount exiting the body. The time required to reach a steady state equals the total of four or five elimination half-lives. Knowing the half-life is important in determining how often a drug should be administered. Drugs with shorter half-lives require more frequent dosing than drugs with longer half-lives.

429. The answer is e. *(Kaplan, 8/e, p 1099.)* Priapism (an abnormally prolonged erection) is estimated to happen in 1 in every 10,000 patients treated with trazodone. The risk for this side effect is higher during the first month of treatment and at low doses. If priapism develops, trazodone should be discontinued immediately and the patient should seek emergency treatment if the erections last for more than 1 h or are significantly painful. The exact cause of trazodone-induced priapism is unknown, but this side effect is thought to be due to an α_1-antagonistic action in the circulatory system of the penis. If untreated, prolonged priapism can cause permanent impotence.

430. The answer is d. *(Kaplan, 8/e, p 1105.)* Although one patient survived an overdose of 10 g of amitriptyline, TCAs are usually fatal at dosages between 2 and 3 grams. The ingestion of 700 to 1400 mg causes moderate to severe toxicity. The TCAs' narrow therapeutic window makes them unsuited for highly suicidal patients unless the medication is dispensed under careful supervision.

431. The answer is b. *(Ebert, pp 304–305.)* Electroconvulsive therapy (ECT) is considered the treatment of first choice in severe psychotic depression and in depressed patients who are refractory to medications or cannot tolerate antidepressant side effects. ECT is also used for the treatment of acute mania, catatonia, neuroleptic malignant syndrome, and Parkinson's disease. ECT has been proven as effective as or superior to all pharmacological agents to which it has been compared. There are no absolute contraindications for ECT. Relative contraindications include a recent myocardial infarct, illnesses that increase intracranial pressure, medical disorders that disrupt the blood-brain barrier, recent cerebrovascular incidents, cerebral aneurysms, and bleeding disorders. ECT is a safe procedure. The risk of death has been estimated at 1 in every 25,000 treatments, which is roughly equivalent to the risk of death in patients exposed to general anesthesia alone.

432. The answer is e. *(Kaplan, 8/e, p 983.)* Cyproheptadine has been used to reverse the negative effects of SSRIs on sexual function. Other medications used for this purpose are yohimbine, bethanechol, amantidine, and bupropion. Bupropion has been reported to increase sex drive, possibly by dopaminergic activity and increased production of norepinephrine.

433. The answer is d. *(Kaplan, 8/e, p 172.)* Double-blind crossover studies are done to control for individual differences in drug response and the placebo effect. The term double-blind refers to the fact that neither the subject nor the researcher knows whether the substance being taken is placebo or drug. The term crossover refers to changing from drug to placebo, or vice versa, in mid-study, without the knowledge of the subject or researcher.

434–435. The answers are 434-b, 435-d. *(Kaplan, 8/e, p 944.)* Dopamine receptor blockade causes hyperprolactinemia, which in turn can cause breast enlargement, galactorrhea (abnormal discharge of milk from the breast), and suppression of testosterone production in men.

436. The answer is c. *(Kaplan, 8/e, p 1052.)* Several nonsteroidal antiinflammatory drugs, including ibuprofen, naproxen, diclofenac, and indomethacin, can increase plasma lithium levels and have been associated with toxicity. The mechanism of action is thought to be an inhibition of renal tubular prostaglandin synthesis.

437. The answer is e. *(Kaplan, 8/e, p 996.)* Triazolam has the shortest average half life (2 h), followed by alprazolam (12 h), lorazepam (15 h), and diazepam and flurazepam (both 100 h). These figures include the half-life of the active metabolites.

438. The answer is d. *(Kaplan, 8/e, p 1021.)* The potency of an antipsychotic describes its relative ability to block postsynaptic dopamine receptors. Haloperidol and fluphenazine are examples of high-potency neuroleptics. Chlorpromazine and thioridazine are low-potency, while perphenazine and molindone are considered to have intermediate potency. The potency of the neuroleptic will effect its therapeutic dosage (effective daily doses of haloperidol are usually between 5 and 20 mg, while chlorpromazine requires dosages of 200 to 600 mg/d). Low- and high-potency neuroleptics also differ in their side effect profiles. In general, the lower-potency medications are more anticholinergic and sedating and are more likely to cause hypotension. The higher-potency medications tend to cause more extrapyramidal side effects.

439. The answer is a. *(Kaplan, 8/e, p 1049.)* Lithium affects thyroid function, and 7 to 9% of patients have been reported to develop hypothyroidism with lithium treatment. About 30% of long-term lithium-treated patients have elevated levels of TSH. If symptoms of hypothyroidism appear, treatment with levothyroxine is indicated.

440. The answer is b. *(Kaplan, 8/e, p 1008–1014.)* Aplastic anemia is a rare, idiosyncratic, non-dose-related side effect of carbamazepine. Stevens-Johnson syndrome is a potentially life-threatening exfoliative dermatitis, also rarely associated with carbamazepine treatment. Neuroleptic malignant syndrome, serotonin syndrome, and malignant hyperthermia are not associated with this medication.

441. The answer is d. *(Kaplan, 8/e, pp 1070–1074.)* Clozapine has been proven effective in a significant percentage of schizophrenic patients refractory to other neuroleptics. Clozapine is also approved for the treatment of patients who experience intolerable extrapyramidal symptoms on other neuroleptics and for the treatment of tardive dyskinesia. Unlike the other typical and atypical neuroleptics (besides olanzapine), clozapine is effective for the positive as well as the negative symptoms of schizophrenia. Due to the risk of agranulocytosis (1 to 2%), clozapine is not approved for patients who can tolerate and benefit from other medications.

442. The answer is d. *(Kaplan, 8/e, p 1089.)* Serotonin syndrome is characterized by abdominal pain, diarrhea, excessive sweating, fever, tachycardia, elevated blood pressure, alteration of mental status including delirium, myoclonus, increased motor activity, and mood changes. In the most severe cases, hyperpyrexia, shock, and death can occur. This syndrome is due to an overactivation of serotoninergic receptors by an excess of serotonin. Serotonin syndrome can develop whenever two serotoninergic medications are combined or during the coadministration of an MAO inhibitor and an SSRI or a tricyclic antidepressant. For this reason, when switching from a TCA or an SSRI to an MAO inhibitor, a washout period of 2 weeks is recommended (5 weeks for fluoxetine, given its long half-life).

443. The answer is a. *(Kaplan, 8/e, p 1072.)* Phenothiazines, tricyclic antidepressants, and antiparkinsonian agents (such as benztropine mesylate) all have anticholinergic properties. The action of these drugs becomes additive when they are administered in combination. It is not uncommon for persons receiving such a combination to show evidence of a mild organic brain syndrome, including difficulty in concentrating; impaired short-term memory; disorientation, which often is more noticeable at night; and dry skin due to inhibition of sweating.

444. The answer is b. *(Kaplan, 8/e, p 454.)* A number of drugs can cause depression. These include several adrenocortical steroids, such as prednisone and cortisone; estrogens and progestins found in birth control pills; thyroid medications; antihypertensive medications; antiparkinsonian medications; and many others. These drugs may cause depression directly or on withdrawal. Ibuprofen, acetylsalicylate, and acetaminophen do not cause depression. Imipramine is used to treat depression.

445. The answer is e. *(Kaplan, 8/e, p 1070.)* Discontinuation of the antipsychotic medication or a dosage decrease are the initial interventions recommended when tardive dyskinesia is first diagnosed. If discontinuation is not possible and dosage decrease is not effective, clozapine has been proved effective in ameliorating and suppressing the symptoms of tardive dyskinesia.

446. The answer is c. *(Kaplan, 8/e, p 1105.)* Tricyclic antidepressants have type I, quinidine-like antiarrhythmic properties. Like quinidine, they have a membrane-stabilizing effect that results in slowing of cardiac conduction, and, at high levels, they cause potentially fatal heart blocks. Since cardiac arrhythmias are the main cause of death following a TCA antidepressant overdose, ECG monitoring is essential. QRS prolongation is the most accurate indicator of the severity of the overdose.

447. The answer is b. *(Ebert, p 273.)* Patients on clozapine must be monitored regularly for the appearance of agranulocytosis, which occurs in 1 to 2% of all patients treated. Erythrocyte and platelet concentrations are unaffected.

448. The answer is b. *(Kaplan, 8/e, p 1019.)* Antipsychotic drugs block dopamine receptor sites. Blockade of dopamine receptors in the limbic system is believed to be responsible for the antipsychotic effects. Blockade in the basal ganglia receptors results in the extrapyramidal symptoms that accompany neuroleptic treatment.

Psychopharmacology and Other Somatic Therapies　　Answers　275

449. The answer is e. *(Kaplan, 8/e, p 1113.)* Carbamazepine and valproate are associated with an increased risk of neural tube defects and spina bifida when they are used during the first trimester of pregnancy. The risk is thought to be higher with valproate. If medications are necessary to treat severe manic symptoms during pregnancy, neuroleptics are usually preferred because there is no conclusive evidence that their use, even in the first trimester, causes fetal malformations.

450. The answer is c. *(Kaplan, 8/e, p 1040.)* Long-acting injectable antipsychotic medications are not used for the treatment of acute psychosis but can be advantageous for the maintenance treatment of patients not compliant with oral medications. Furthermore, since the variation of drug absorption and the effects of first-pass hepatic metabolism are bypassed, drug concentrations may be more consistent with depot preparations. In the United States, haloperidol decanoate, fluphenazine decanoate, and fluphenazine enanthate are the only antipsychotics available in injectable depot form. Maintenance doses for long-acting fluphenazine range from 12.5 to 50 mg intramuscularly every 2 weeks. For haloperidol decanoate, the effective dose range is between 25 and 200 mg intramuscularly every 4 weeks.

451. The answer is e. *(Kaplan, 8/e, p 1103.)* Urinary retention, blurred vision, constipation, and dry mouth are common anticholinergic side effects associated with tricyclic antidepressants. Among these medications, amitriptyline has the most powerful atropinic properties. Venlafaxine, bupropion, trazodone, and nefazodone do not have significant anticholinergic effects.

452. The answer is b. *(Kaplan, 8/e, pp 1089–1090.)* Fluoxetine inhibits the metabolism of several drugs, including carbamazepine, diazepam, and haloperidol. Because it is metabolized by CYP 2D6, fluoxetine may interfere with the metabolism of other drugs in the small percentage of the patient population who are poor metabolizers.

453. The answer is e. *(Kaplan, 8/e, p 1015.)* Dopamine antagonists are effective in reducing the symptoms of Tourette's disorder in 60 to 70% of cases. Haloperidol and pimozide are the most commonly used, but other antipsychotics including fluphenazine and risperidone have proven to be effective in open clinical trials. Clonidine may also be used to avoid the serious side effects associated with the neuroleptics. Amphetamines, such as methylphenidate, may exacerbate tics.

454. The answer is c. *(Kaplan, 8/e, pp 1220–1221.)* Haloperidol is the most frequently prescribed drug for Tourette's disorder. Almost 80% of patients have a good response, with their symptom frequency and severity decreasing by 70 to 90%. However, studies indicate that only 20 to 30% of patients stay on haloperidol for long-term maintenance, probably due to the medication's adverse side effects.

455. The answer is e. *(Kaplan, 8/e, p 943.)* Depression in elderly persons, especially those who already have some evidence of dementia, may present with a worsening of cognitive functions (pseudodementia). Differentiating progressing dementia from depression may be difficult. If the onset of symptoms is reasonably abrupt (1 or 2 months) and the patient has other signs suggestive of depression (e.g., changes in sleeping and eating habits accompanied by motor retardation or agitation), depression should be considered. It certainly is preferable to consider a trial of antidepressants, which might be beneficial, rather than to assume a person's dementia is progressive and untreatable. Among the antidepressants, SSRIs such as sertraline are preferred to TCAs because they lack anticholinergic and cardiotoxic side effects and do not cause orthostatic hypotension.

456–457. The answers are 456-b, 457-e. *(Kaplan, 8/e, pp 1018–1019.)* Disulfiram inhibits acetaldehyde dehydrogenase, one of the main enzymes in the metabolism of ethyl alcohol. Ingestion of alcohol, even in small quantities, causes accumulation of toxic acetaldehyde and a variety of unpleasant symptoms, including facial flushing, tachycardia, vomiting, and nausea. Many over-the-counter cough and cold medications contain as much as 40% alcohol and can precipitate such a reaction. The intensity of the disulfiram-alcohol interaction varies with each patient and with the quantity of alcohol consumed. Extreme cases are characterized by respiratory depression, seizures, cardiovascular collapse, and even death. For this reason, the use of disulfiram is recommended only with highly motivated patients who will agree to carefully avoid any food or medication containing alcohol.

458. The answer is c. *(Kaplan, 8/e, p 1093.)* There is no cure for narcolepsy, but stimulants such as methylphenidate, pemoline, and amphetamine can ameliorate daytime sleepiness. Medications that reduce REM sleep, such as TCAs and SSRIs, are used if cataplexy is also present.

459. The answer is d. *(Kaplan, 8/e, pp 1070–1074.)* Clozapine is the preferred treatment for psychotic symptoms in patients with Parkinson's disease. Due to its relative sparing of the nigrostriatal dopaminergic system and its anticholinergic effects, clozapine does not worsen and may in fact ameliorate Parkinsonian symptoms. Typical antipsychotic medications, on the contrary, tend to aggravate the extrapyramidal symptoms of patients with Parkinson's.

460. The answer is c. *(Kaplan, 8/e, pp 567–571.)* If there is no change in symptomatology after 3 to 4 weeks of treatment at an adequate dosage, another antidepressant should be considered. If there is a partial response, the trial should be continued for another 2 or 3 weeks. In this case, the patient is on a somewhat low dosage of sertraline, which should be increased for another several weeks before a decision is made to change to another medication or augment it.

461. The answer is a. *(Kaplan, 8/e, p 1051.)* A pregnancy test is necessary before initiating lithium treatment because this medication has been associated with congenital malformations. The most common anomalies reportedly associated with lithium are cardiovascular, especially Ebstein's anomaly (i.e., a congenital downward displacement of a distorted tricuspid valve into the right ventricle). Recent studies have found that the early studies may have overestimated this risk markedly. While it is still ideal for pregnant women to be completely free of drug use of any kind, the continuation of lithium therapy should not be completely ruled out.

462. The answer is c. *(Kaplan, 8/e, pp 1046–1047.)* Since the half-life of lithium is about 20 h, equilibrium is reached after 5 to 7 days of regular intake. (Steady state is reached after approximately 5 half-lives of the drug being administered.)

463. The answer is b. *(Kaplan, 8/e, pp 973–978.)* Propranolol and other beta blockers, taken 1 h before public speaking or other events that can trigger performance anxiety, reduce symptoms of sympathetic activity such as tremor, tachycardia, and sweating that may serve as cues for reinforcing anxiety and fear. Since beta receptor blockade causes bronchospasm, these medications are contraindicated in patients with asthma. One might consider the use of selective beta blockers for patients with bronchospasm (i.e., atenolol and metoprolol).

464. The answer is d. *(Kaplan, 8/e, p 1096.)* The connection between thyroid function and mood disorders has been known for more than a century, since nineteenth-century physicians noticed that hypothyroidism was accompanied by depression. All the hormones of the hypothalamic-pituitary-thyroid axis have been used in the treatment of depression, alone or in combination with other agents, although the most commonly used are liothyronine and levothyroxine.

465. The answer is e. *(Kaplan, 8/e, p 1107.)* Approximately 5 to 10% of Caucasian individuals metabolize nortriptyline and desipramine at a much slower rate than the general population, due to an inherited deficiency of the P 450 isozyme 2D6. These individuals, known as poor metabolizers, develop toxic levels at very low medication doses.

466. The answer is e. *(Kaplan, 8/e, p 1072.)* The occurrence of seizures during clozapine treatment is dose-related and increases considerably with dosages greater than 400 mg/d. Phenobarbitol is considered the safest and the best-tolerated anticonvulsivant for patients taking clozapine who experience seizures. It should be started after clozapine is stopped; then the clozapine can be restarted at 50% of its previous dosage and then gradually raised. Carbamazepine should be avoided because the bone marrow suppression risk of this medication can increase clozapine's risk for agranulocytosis.

467. The answer is a. *(Kaplan, 8/e, p 1123.)* Patients with seasonal depression and bipolar depression with a seasonal component can benefit from exposure to bright light, in the range of 1,500 to 10,000 lux or more for 1 to 2 h every day before dawn. Phototherapy is effective alone in mild cases and as an adjunct to medication treatment in more severe cases.

468. The answer is a. *(Kaplan, 8/e, p 993.)* Practically every class of medication has been used to treat posttraumatic stress disorder, including every family of antidepressant, mood stabilizers; anxiolytics; and inhibitors of adrenergic activity, such as clonidine and propanolol. Clonidine and beta blockers can be particularly useful, alone or in combination with other medications, to treat symptoms of hyperarousal.

469. The answer is d. *(Kaplan, 8/e, p 1038.)* High-potency neuroleptics, such as haloperidol and fluphenazine, being low in anticholinergic side effects and less likely to cause postural hypotension, are preferred to low-potency medications such as chlorpromazine in elderly patients with cardiovascular problems and prostatic hypertrophy. Clozapine is not recommended due to its powerful anticholinergic effects, its tendency to cause hypotension, and its risk for agranulocytosis. Thioridazine is the least appropriate medication in this case because, aside from sharing the side effects profile of the other low-potency neuroleptics, it can cause fatal arrhythmias by prolonging the QT interval. Finally, olanzapine is not appropriate in this patient because it causes significant postural hypotension.

470. The answer is c. *(Kaplan, 8/e, p 1089.)* Abrupt discontinuation of an SSRI causes a variety of symptoms that can be quite distressing for the patient. The most common physical symptoms are dizziness, nausea, vomiting, lethargy, flulike symptoms (chills and aches), and sensory and sleep disturbances. Commonly reported psychological symptoms are irritability, anxiety, and crying spells. Symptoms usually emerge 1 to 3 days after the last dose. Paroxetine and sertraline, due to their shorter half-life, are the SSRIs most likely to cause a discontinuation syndrome and should be tapered over several weeks. Due to its long half-life and its active metabolites, fluoxetine can be stopped abruptly without problems.

471. The answer is a. *(Kaplan, 8/e, p 989.)* Benzodiazepines bind to GABA receptors, which represent the main cortical and thalamic inhibitory system, and potentiate the response of these receptors to GABA. Benzodiazepines do not have any direct effect on the GABA receptors unless GABA is present.

472–473. The answers are 472-a, 473-a. *(Kaplan, 8/e, p 1062.)* Over-the-counter medications containing sympathomimetic agents such as pseudoephedrine can cause severe hypertensive crises in patients on MAOIs due to the inhibition of their main metabolic pathway. Tyramine, a powerful hypertensive agent, is contained in many foods and is usually metabolized by monoamine oxidase. Foods to be avoided by patients on MAOIs include tyramine-rich foods such as aged cheese, salami, sausage, overripe fruit, liquors, red wine, pickled fish, sauerkraut, and brewer's yeast. Chocolate, coffee, tea, beer, and white wine can be consumed in small quantities.

474. The answer is d. *(Kaplan, 8/e, p 1093.)* Many antidepressants, including SSRIs, TCAs, and MAOIs, suppress REM sleep and can be useful in the treatment of cataplexy. The other medications listed do not affect sleep cycles.

475. The answer is d. *(Ebert, p 158.)* Neuroleptic malignant syndrome (NMS) is a relatively rare but potentially fatal complication of neuroleptic treatment. Its main features are hyperthermia, severe muscular rigidity, autonomic instability, and changes in mental status. Associated findings are increased CPK, increased liver transaminase activity, leukocytes, and myoglobinuria. The mortality rate can be as high as 30% and can be higher when the syndrome is precipitated by depot forms. Neuroleptic malignant syndrome is more common in young males when high-potency neuroleptics are used in high doses and when dosage is escalated rapidly.

476. The answer is a. *(Ebert, p 158.)* The first step in management of NMS is discontinuation of all antipsychotic medications. Supportive treatments include treatment of extrapyramidal symptoms with antiparkinson medications, correcting fluid imbalances, treating fever, and managing hypertension or hypotension. Dopaminergic agents such as dantrolene, bromocriptine, and amantidine are used in the treatment of more severe cases.

477. The answer is e. *(Ebert, p 541.)* Imipramine is effective in the treatment of nocturnal enuresis, through a still unknown mechanism. Its beneficial effects in this disorder may be related to its anticholinergic properties or an effect on the sleep process. Imipramine is also used with good results in the treatment of children and adults with ADHD, although it is not as effective as the stimulants. Imipramine can be helpful in patients with comorbid anxiety or tics, patients who do not tolerate stimulants, or patients who have a history of substance abuse.

478. The answer is d. *(Kaplan, 8/e, pp 968–973.)* The use of acetylcholinesterase inhibitors in Alzheimer's disease is based on the observation that this disorder is characterized by a massive loss of cholinergic neurons. Direct cholinergic stimulation has not been effective in the treatment of dementia, but several cholinesterase inhibitors such as tacrine, donepezil, metrifonate, and galantamine have been effective in improving the cognitive functions of Alzheimer's patients in the short term. These drugs have not proven as effective in the long term, however.

479. The answer is b. *(Kaplan, 8/e, pp 1053–1054.)* The lithium level considered effective for acute mania is between 1 and 1.5 meq/L. Levels above 1.5 meq/L carry a risk of toxicity that outweighs the potential benefits. Lithium levels need to be interpreted in the context of the clinical presentation, because some patients, especially the medically ill and the elderly, may present with clear symptoms of lithium toxicity at levels below 1.5 meq/L.

480. The answer is b. *(Kaplan, 8/e, p 1104.)* Tricyclic antidepressants have a quinidine-like antiarrhythmic effect and slow cardiac conduction. Although at therapeutic dosages they may have a beneficial effect on ventricular excitability, in patients with preexisting prolonged QRS or in any person at toxic dosages, TCAs can cause a fatal heart block. TCAs do not affect cardiac contractility or cardiac output, nor do they cause cardiomyopathy or valvular deformities.

481–484. The answers are 481-h, 482-d, 483-a, 484-g. *(Kaplan, 8/e, pp 881, 1031, 1032, 1049.)* Lithium causes a benign, high-frequency, fine tremor that worsens during activities requiring fine motor control. Dose reduction, elimination of caffeine, slow-release lithium preparations, and beta blockers are the main therapeutic interventions. A severe tremor at any time during lithium treatment may be a sign of toxicity. Neuroleptic-induced dystonia is characterized by intermittent or sustained muscle spasms, usually involving the head and neck. Common symptoms include torticollis (neck spasms), tongue spasms that interfere with speech, and oculogyric crises (eyes forced in an upward gaze). Opisthotonus can also occur but is less frequent. Dystonic reactions are more common in young males, at the beginning of the treatment, and when high-potency neuroleptics are used. Anticholinergic medications such as benztropine and diphenhydramine, administered intramuscularly, are the treatments of choice. Coarse, pill-rolling, nonintentional tremor that improves with intentional movement and worsens at rest is characteristic of Parkinson's disease and neuroleptic-induced parkinsonism. Cogwheel rigidity, a stiff gait with short steps, and expressionless face and speech are other common Parkinsonian symptoms. Rabbit syndrome is an uncommon extrapyramidal neuroleptic-induced syndrome often confused with tardive dyskinesia. In this syndrome, the chewing movements are much more rapid and regular than the orofacial choreoathetoid movements typical of tardive dyskinesia. Furthermore, the tongue and other parts of the body are not involved.

Law and Ethics in Psychiatry

Questions

DIRECTIONS: Each item below contains a question or incomplete statement followed by suggested responses. Select the **one best** response to each question.

485. In order to successfully sue for medical malpractice, a plaintiff must prove four elements. Three of these elements are negligent performance of patient care, harm to the patient as a direct result of the physician's actions, and damage or harm to the patient. Which of the following is the fourth element?

a. The patient was not informed of the actions the physician was taking
b. The patient was not in agreement with the treatment plan
c. Notes were not kept in an orderly and complete fashion
d. There was a duty on the part of the physician to treat the patient
e. There was intent to harm the patient

486. A 56-year-old woman in the last stages of amyotrophic lateral sclerosis asks for her life support to be stopped and to be allowed to die. Her family members disagree with her decision and go to court to keep the patient alive. A psychiatric evaluation finds the patient mentally sound and fully able to understand the consequences of her decision. Referring to the Supreme Court's decision on the Cruzan v. Director case, which of the following rulings is decided on by the court?

a. The family's desires overrule the patient's wishes
b. Terminating one's life is illegal
c. A guardian must be appointed to make decisions on behalf of the patient
d. Since the patient's life expectancy is more than two weeks, she cannot be allowed to die
e. The patient is competent, and as such she has the right to refuse unwanted medical treatment

Items 487–488

487. An emaciated 26-year-old man is brought to the emergency room by the local police late one night in the dead of winter. The police tell the psychiatrist on call that the man was preaching loudly at a nearby busy intersection, sometimes walking into traffic to approach drivers while dressed only in a thin robe despite the freezing temperatures. On interview, the psychiatrist notes that the man displays delusions of special connections to God and discounts any concern for his physical safety as he will leave his fate to God. The patient refuses voluntary admission, stating that he must get back to his divine mission. On what grounds would the emergency room psychiatrist be most justified in hospitalizing the patient involuntarily?

a. The patient is so disorganized as to be unable to attend to his basic physical needs
b. The patient is suffering from acute psychosis
c. The patient is at risk for causing harm to other people
d. The patient's psychiatric disorder is likely to worsen in the future without treatment
e. The patient's behavior could be interpreted as actively suicidal

488. The patient in question 487 is admitted to the hospital involuntarily. On the inpatient unit, he is noted to be mild-mannered and soft-spoken. He refuses all forms of treatment, stating that God is his only healer. While the patient is not particularly disruptive and not aggressive in any way, staff are nevertheless concerned about his refusal of treatment. In fact, he is noted to be trying very persistently to "convert" the other patients and staff on the unit, sometimes to their marked irritation. A decision is made by the staff to medicate the patient against his will. Subsequently, members of the patient's family bring suit against the clinical team working with the patient. On what grounds would the lawsuit initiated by the family most likely be brought?

a. The involuntary treatment violated the family's constitutional rights
b. The treatment violated the family's religious beliefs
c. The patient had a right to refuse treatment because he was not in any immediate danger
d. The treatment could have caused side effects
e. The patient did not have a history of aggressive behavior

489. The family of a 49-year-old chronic schizophrenic male brings a lawsuit against the community mental health center where he has been treated for the past 14 years. They express concern that the patient has developed some persistent chewing movements of his mouth, over which he appears to have no control. On what grounds would such a lawsuit most likely be successful?

a. The patient had not been given adequate disclosure of the risks and benefits of his treatment
b. The patient received improper medication
c. The patient received excessively high doses of medications
d. The family had not given informed consent for the treatment
e. The doctors had not told the family that the treatment was potentially harmful

490. Which of the following statements constitutes the standard for legal insanity in U.S. federal courts?

a. Lack of capacity, because of a mental illness, to appreciate the wrongfulness of conduct or to conform conduct to the requirements of the law
b. A crime that was the product of the defendant's mental illness, whether or not the person understands that what he did was wrong
c. Severe psychosis during the criminal act
d. Mental incapacity to have performed the required criminal intent
e. The lack of substantial capacity to appreciate the right from wrong

491. Which of the following statements best defines the term "privileged communication"?

a. Psychiatrists have the privilege of disclosing information about a patient to other psychiatrists, mental health professionals, or physicians
b. The information revealed by psychiatrists at a probate hearing is handled as privileged
c. Psychiatrists are granted by the court the privilege of disclosing information about a specific patient
d. Patients have the statutory right to prevent psychiatrists from disclosing confidential information
e. Psychiatrists can reveal some but not all information

492. The landmark decision in Tarasoff-I held that a therapist has an obligation to do which of the following?
a. Protect the confidentiality of information obtained during therapy
b. Notify the police when a patient is involved in illegal activities
c. Report a minor's sexual activity to the patient's parents
d. Warn the potential victim of a potentially violent patient
e. Seek informed consent from patients who are given neuroleptic medications

493. Which of the following is the most common cause of malpractice claims in psychiatric practice?
a. Improper treatment resulting in physical injury
b. Homicide
c. Sexual involvement between physician and patient
d. Failure to treat psychosis
e. Improper certification in hospitalization

494. A patient with a family history of Huntington's disease wishes to select his nephew as the person to make decisions about his health care if he should become incompetent. Which of the following documents will need to be used?
a. Last testament
b. Durable power of attorney
c. Informed consent
d. Competency evaluation
e. Contract

495. Which of the following statements refers to the principle of beneficence?
a. Prevent harm and promote well-being
b. Do no harm
c. Treat indigent patients without monetary compensation
d. Provide universal health care
e. Build the patient-doctor relationship on trust

496. In Tarasoff-II, the second decision by the California Supreme Court on the case, the original Tarasoff ruling was revised by the addition of which of the following?
a. Requiring the warning of only identifiable potential victims
b. Imposing legal liability on police
c. Requiring hospitalization of patients deemed dangerous
d. Instituting a duty to protect potential victims, not just warn them
e. Requiring use of neuroleptic medication to treat potentially dangerous patients

497. A male psychiatrist and his patient fall in love. The psychiatrist terminates treatment, and they begin a sexual relationship. Which of the following statements about the relevant moral and legal issues for the psychiatrist is true?
a. He is not in violation of the American Psychiatric Association's guidelines for ethical conduct
b. He is not liable to malpractice suits
c. He is not in jeopardy of having his license revoked
d. He is not possibly liable for prosecution for rape
e. If a malpractice suit were ever brought against him, his malpractice insurance would not likely cover any liability incurred

DIRECTIONS: Each group of questions below consists of lettered options followed by a set of numbered items. For each numbered item, select the **one** lettered option with which it is **most** closely associated. Each lettered option may be used once, more than once, or not at all.

Items 498–500

Match each statement to the appropriate legal concept.

a. M'Naghten rule
b. Irresistible impulse rule
c. American Law Institute: Model Penal Code
d. Durham rule
e. Mens rea elements

498. Psychiatric testimony should be addressed only for the issue of state of mind and criminal intent at the time of the crime. **(CHOOSE 1 CONCEPT)**

499. An accused is not criminally responsible if the unlawful act was the product of mental disease or mental defect. **(CHOOSE 1 CONCEPT)**

500. The defendant must have the volition (freedom of will) to refrain from the criminal act. **(CHOOSE 1 CONCEPT)**

Law and Ethics in Psychiatry

Answers

485. The answer is d. *(Kaplan, 8/e, pp 1317–1318.)* In a malpractice lawsuit, the plaintiff must show by a preponderance of evidence that the four elements of malpractice are present. These are the so-called **four D's of malpractice:** (1) a **d**uty existed toward the patient on the part of the psychiatrist; (2) a **d**eviation from the standard of practice occurred; (3) this **d**eviation bore a direct causal relationship to the untoward outcome; and (4) **d**amages occurred as a result.

486. The answer is e. *(Kaplan, 8/e, p 1326.)* Nancy Cruzan had been in a vegetative state, kept alive by feeding tubes, for over 4 years. Because her prognosis was hopeless, her parents went to court to have the feeding stopped so that she could die. The case ultimately found its way to the Supreme Court, which ruled that competent persons have a constitutional right to refuse unwanted medical treatment. The court left it to the states to decide how to handle the situation of the incompetent patient, and, in many states, that has limited the rights of families to make decisions unless there is an advance directive such as a living will or a durable power of attorney.

487. The answer is a. *(Kaplan, 8/e, p 1309.)* The emergency room psychiatrist was justified in hospitalizing the patient involuntarily because the patient appeared to be mentally ill and unable to care for his own basic needs. In this case, being properly clothed to avoid the potential harmful effects of exposure to cold would be considered a basic need. The essential criteria that must be met in order for an involuntary hospitalization to be justified are as follows: there must be evidence of the presence of mental illness; the patient must be at risk for causing imminent harm to him- or herself or to others; and the patient must be unable to provide for his or her basic needs. In the absence of strong evidence for imminent danger or risk of harm to self or others, patients maintain the right to refuse treatment, even when they have been hospitalized involuntarily.

488. The answer is c. *(Kaplan, 8/e, p 1309.)* Since the patient was residing on a hospital unit at the time the unwanted treatments were administered, he was at no immediate risk of the sort that originally led to his admission. Nor was there any evidence that he was acting in ways that placed himself or others in immediate danger or risk of harm. The family's beliefs and rights are not relevant in this context.

489. The answer is a. *(Kaplan, 8/e, p 1312.)* No patient may be treated against his or her own will, nor may any treatments be administered without the patient's having made a truly informed decision about the treatment. In this case, if it was believed that the patient was not capable of making an informed decision about the treatment at the time of its institution, an evaluation of competency should have been conducted and a substituted judgment sought. While cases have been brought against physicians for treating patients with the wrong medication or too high a dose, in this case the use of an antipsychotic was probably appropriate, and tardive dyskinesia can and does occur at appropriate doses.

490. The answer is a. *(Kaplan, 8/e, p 1314.)* Most U.S. federal courts presently use the American Law Institute (ALI) test, or a minor variation, to determine criminal responsibility. The ALI standard states, "It shall be a defense that the defendant at the time of the proscribed conduct, as a result of mental disease or defect, lacked substantial capacity either to appreciate the wrongfulness of his conduct or to conform his conduct to the requirements of the law." Many jurisdictions have appended a section that states, "The terms mental disease or defect do not include an abnormality manifested only by repeated criminal or otherwise antisocial conduct." This provision is designed to prevent persons with antisocial personalities from offering an insanity defense.

491. The answer is d. *(Kaplan, 8/e, p 1306.)* Privileged communication must be provided by statute. Where the privilege exists, it is essentially "owned" by the person whose medical information is being sought. Persons may waive the privilege and allow their psychiatrists to testify. Because there are many qualifications to statutory privilege, some feel that the concept is almost meaningless.

492. The answer is d. *(Kaplan, 8/e, p 1308.)* The Tarasoff decision was a landmark case in determining that psychotherapists have an obligation to warn third parties who are in danger. In this instance, the therapist had an obligation to warn the potential victim of a student who had threatened to kill the girl who had rejected him. The patient ultimately killed the girl, thus prompting the litigation.

493. The answer is a. *(Kaplan, 8/e, pp 1317–1318.)* Improper treatment is the most common reason for malpractice claims in psychiatry, accounting for 33% of all claims. This is followed by attempted or completed suicide, which account for 20% of all claims.

494. The answer is b. *(Kaplan, 8/e, p 1313.)* Patients are increasingly aware and concerned about who will make decisions for them if they lose the ability to make their own decisions due to a recurrent mental illness such as bipolar disorder, a medical illness, or later-life vegetative states. The durable power of attorney allows the selection in advance of a decision maker who can then act without the necessity of a court proceeding.

495. The answer is a. *(Kaplan, 8/e, p 1321.)* The principle of beneficence refers to preventing or removing harm and promoting well-being. This principle, along with that of nonmaleficence (doing no harm), has been until recently the primary driving force behind medical and psychiatric practice throughout history. Now economic considerations figure much more prominently than ever before in clinical decision making. The fiduciary principle states that the doctor-patient relationship is built on a sense of honor and trust that the doctor will act competently and responsibly in partnership with the patient and with the patient's consent. This trust is earned and maintained by continuous attention to the patient's needs, a concept known as responsibility.

496. The answer is d. *(Kaplan, 8/e, p 1308–1309.)* Tarasoff-I held that psychotherapists and the police have a duty to warn third parties who are in danger. Tarasoff-II stated that once a therapist has reasonably determined that a patient poses a serious danger of violence to others, he or she "bears a duty to exercise reasonable care to protect the foreseeable victim of that danger." This is an expansion of the more narrow duty to warn; it also exempted the police from liability. There is no explicit requirement for specific treatment, such as medications or hospitalization, though these might well be employed by the psychiatrist in the management of potentially violent persons.

497. The answer is e. *(Kaplan, 8/e, p 1323.)* In "The Principles of Medical Ethics with Annotations Especially Applicable to Psychiatry," the American Psychiatric Association (APA) unequivocally states that sexual activity with patients is unethical. Such activity is viewed as a misuse and exploitation of the transference relationship, which may activate sexual feelings in both patient and therapist. Psychiatrists have been prosecuted for rape in a few instances, loss of licensure or other licensure action is not uncommon, and malpractice suits with substantial settlements are increasingly common. While some have advocated that a waiting period of a year might be a reasonable way to approach this ethical issue, the APA has pointed out that the transference may persist long after treatment ends. Insurance carriers for the APA and the American Medical Association (AMA) exclude liability for any such sexual activity.

498–500. The answers are 498-e, 499-d, 500-b. *(Kaplan, 8/e, pp 1315, 1317.)* The AMA has recommended, and some states have codified, that the insanity defense be abolished. There is considerable question as to whether this can be done constitutionally. Such attempts often direct that the psychiatrist should testify only as to the mens rea elements in criminal trials. This is testimony that addresses the issue of whether the defendant possessed a criminal intent or state of mind at the time of the crime. The Durham rule, a 1954 decision by the District of Columbia Circuit Court, eliminated the cognitive issues that were associated with the M'Naghten rule, as well as the concept of irresistible impulse that had expanded it in some jurisdictions in order to introduce the concept of volitional control over one's behavior. It gave wide latitude to psychiatric testimony. It was rejected in 1972 because there was simply too much variation in psychiatric opinion as to what constituted the product of mental disease or mental defect. Most federal circuit courts and approximately 25 states have adopted at least parts of the rule developed by the ALI. The rule has at least some elements of cognitive (M'Naghten) and volitional (irresistible impulse) determinations. However, it is no longer an issue of all or nothing. The word *appreciate,* for example, acknowledges that a psychotic person may know right from wrong, but may lack an ability to truly comprehend the substance and consequences of the behavior. Consider the case of a psychotic who knows that murder is morally and legally wrong, but who kills a neighbor while acting under the influence of paranoid delusions and compelling hallucinations. In 1843, Daniel M'Naghten was accused of killing the secretary of the prime minister of Great

Britain. He was acquitted on grounds of insanity, and public outrage led to the development of the M'Naghten test regarding criminal insanity. It is a test primarily related to cognitive functions. It became the test of insanity in many jurisdictions in the United States and is still retained by some states. The Model Penal Code developed by the American Law Institute (ALI) did not attempt to define mental disease or defect, but it did specify that "the terms 'mental disease' or 'defect' do not include an abnormality manifested only by repeated criminal or otherwise antisocial conduct." This reflected the opinion that sociopaths should not be able to evade criminal responsibility for their acts by claiming that their behavior was on the basis of their psychiatric problem.

Bibliography

Ebert MH, Loosen PT, Nurcombe B (eds): *Current Diagnosis and Treatment in Psychiatry.* New York, Lange/McGraw-Hill, 2000.

Goldman HH: *Review of General Psychiatry,* 5/e. New York, Lange/McGraw-Hill, 2000.

Hales RE, Yudofsky SC (eds): *The American Psychiatric Publishing Textbook of Clinical Psychiatry,* 4/e. Washington, DC: American Psychiatric Press, 2002.

Harrison's Online: www.harrisonline.com.

Kaplan HI, Sadock BJ: *Synopsis of Psychiatry: Behavioral Sciences/Clinical Psychiatry.* 8/e. Philadelphia, Lippincott Williams & Wilkins, 1998.

Stoudemire A: *Clinical Psychiatry for Medical Students,* 3/e. Philadelphia, Lippincott Williams & Wilkins, 1998.

Index

A
Abreaction, 163
Absorption, 168
Abstinence, as Freudian concept, 159, 172
Abstract thinking, 8, 22–23, 27
Acetaldehyde dehydrogenase, 238, 246, 260, 276
Acethylcholine, 75
Acetylcholinesterase inhibitors, 267, 280–281
Acting out, 39, 53–55
Adjustment disorders, 210, 223
Affect
  incongruent, 12, 26, 27
  isolation of, 152, 166
Aggression
  from Amok, 145
  and serotonin levels, 64, 75
Agoraphobia, 198, 204, 205
Agranulocytosis, 142, 257, 274, 278
Akathisia, 249, 269
Alcohol, 260, 276
  dependence, 234, 235, 243–244
  intoxication, 233, 242, 243
  tolerance, 236, 245
  use during pregnancy, 81, 86
  withdrawal, 234, 242, 243
Alcoholism
  and depression, 183, 191
  inheritance of, 237, 246
Aldehyde dehydrogenase, 244
Altruism, 158, 171
Alzheimer's disease, 91, 96, 108–110, 113, 114, 122, 191
  acetylcholinesterase inhibitors for treating, 280–281

Amantadine, 138
American Law Institute (ALI), 292
  and Model Penal Code, 293
  test for criminal responsibility, 285, 290
Amitriptyline, 275
Amnesia
  dissociative, 195, 203
  retrograde, 74
Amok, 136, 145
Amphetamines, 237, 245, 276, 277
  psychosis from, 134, 144
Amylase, serum levels of, 17
Anal stage, 42, 55, 56
Anhedonia, 28
Anonymity, as Freudian concept, 172
Anorexia nervosa, 92, 110
Anticholinergic syndrome, 256, 273–274
Anticonvulsants, 59, 70, 278
  for treating mania, 186
Antidepressants, 179, 188
  and REM sleep suppression, 265, 280
Antisocial personality disorder, 72, 212, 213, 224, 290
Anxiety, 17, 72, 90, 167–168, 173
  performance, 204
  separation, 82, 87–88
  stranger, 36–37, 51
Anxiety disorders, 18, 115–116, 171
Apraxia, 21
Arbitrary inference, 165
Archetypes, 34, 50
Arsenic poisoning, 101, 118
Asceticism, 172
Attachment
  insecure, 44
  secure, 31, 44

Index

Attention-deficit/hyperactivity disorder (ADHD), 79, 85, 250, 270
   imipramine for treating, 280
Autism, 84, 90, 222
Autistic phase, 45
Autonomy vs. shame and doubt, 46, 48
Autoscopic psychosis, 137, 146
Aversive stimulus, 167
Avoidant personality disorder, 171, 215, 222
   contrasted with social phobia, 226

B

Barbiturates, 245
Basic trust, 44
Beck, cognitive model of, 181, 189
Beck Depression Inventory (BDI), 183, 191
Behavioral analysis, 153, 167
Behavioral therapy, 80, 85–86, 157, 165, 168, 170
Benzodiazepines, 187, 203, 206
   and GABA receptors, 265, 279
   half-life of, 254, 272
   for treating alcohol withdrawal delirium, 243
   for treating PCP intoxication, 236, 245
Beta blockers, 200, 206, 279
   and asthma, 262, 278
   for treating akathisia, 249, 269
Biofeedback, 156, 169–170
Biogenic amines, 66, 76
Bipolar disorder, 18, 141, 142, 177, 186
Black-and-white thinking, 165
Blocking, 13, 27
Body dysmorphic disorder, 11, 25, 118, 199, 205
Borderline personality disorder, 10, 18, 24, 94, 112, 118, 147, 161, 171, 188
   psychoanalytic theories of, 211, 223–224

Bowlby, John, theories of, 31, 42, 44, 55, 173, 181, 189
Brain
   damage to, 60, 67, 71, 77
   tumors of, 105, 106, 110, 113, 121
Brief individual psychotherapy, 157, 158, 170
Brief psychotic disorder, 133, 143
Broca's aphasia, 68, 74, 77
Bromocriptine, 125, 138
Bulimia nervosa, 17
Buproprion, 188, 271
Buspirone, 196, 203, 204

C

Caffeine, withdrawal, 235, 244
California verbal learning test, 21
Cannabis, 238, 246
   use during pregnancy, 86
Capgras syndrome, 146
Carbamazepine, side effects of, 145, 255, 273, 275, 278
Case management, 25
Catalepsy, 28
Cataplexy, 59, 70
Catatonia, posturing with, 6–7, 21, 140
Catecholamines, 66, 76
Caudate nucleus, 69, 78
Cerebrovascular disease, depression with, 178, 186–187
Child abuse, 82, 88
   sexual, 211, 223–224
Childhood depression, 83, 89, 182, 190
Childhood disintegrative disorder, 18
Chlordiazepoxide, 243
Chlorpromazine, 131, 142, 272
Chronic traumatic encephalopathy, 108, 123
Circadian sleep disorder, 218, 228
Circumstantiality, 1, 13, 16, 26, 27
Clarification, 168

Client-centered psychotherapy, 150, 164
Clomipramine, 250, 270
Clonidine, 235, 244, 276, 279
Clouding of consciousness, 16
Clozapine, 130, 141, 142, 257, 270, 279
  for Parkinson's disease, 261, 277
  for schizophrenia, 255, 273
  and seizures, 263, 278
  and TD, 256, 274
Cocaine, 62, 73, 236, 245
  dementia from, 92, 109
  intoxication, 237, 245–246
  use during pregnancy, 86–87
Cognitive-behavioral techniques, 204
Cognitive restructuring, 162
Cognitive therapy, 148, 151, 162, 165
Cohort studies, 64, 75
Cold turkey, 241
Compulsions, 14, 28, 202
Computed tomography (CT), 23
Concrete operational stage, 45
Concrete thinking, 4, 19, 22–23
Condensation, 40, 54, 57
Conditioned stimulus, 167
Conduct disorder, 84, 90
Confrontation, 168
Conscious, 56–57
Conversion disorder, 10, 24, 93, 110, 194, 201–202
Coprophilia, 229
Cotard syndrome, 146
Counterconditioning, 168
Countertransference, 7, 22, 150, 164
Creatinine phosphokinase (CPK) levels, 107, 122, 280
Creutzfeldt-Jakob disease, 97, 114, 115
Cross-dressing, 215, 222, 226
Cruzan v. Director case, 283, 289
Cushing's syndrome, 112, 121
Cyclothymic disorder, 180, 188
Cyproheptadine, 252, 271

D

Dantrolene, 138
Defense mechanisms, 38, 52–53, 152, 153, 157, 158, 166–167, 170–172
Delirium, 8, 17, 19, 23
  polypharmacy, 104, 120
  postcardiotomy, 104, 121
Delirium tremens, 234, 243
Delusional disorder, 128, 140–142
Delusions, 1, 16, 17, 53, 132, 143
  in schizophrenia, 139
  somatic, 111, 139
Dementia, 2, 17, 276
Denial, 152, 153, 166
Dependence, defined, 248
Dependent personality disorder, 212, 224
Depersonalization, 22, 28, 197, 204–205
Depression, 17, 111, 112, 189
  from adrenocortical steroids, 256, 274
  with alcoholism, 183, 191
  atypical, 183, 184, 192
  with cerebrovascular disease, 178, 186–187
  in children, 83, 89, 182, 190
  double, 183, 184, 191–192
  in elderly, 259, 276
  major, 60, 61, 71, 73, 127, 139, 175, 185–187
  melancholic, 183, 184, 191
  with MS, 113
  with oral contraceptive use, 180, 188
  psychotic, 177, 186
  seasonal, 263, 278
Depressive position, 46
Derealization, 14, 27
Dereistic thinking, 28
Desensitization, 154, 167–168, 173
Devaluation, 172
Dhat, 145
Diagnostic axes, 15, 29, 225
Diazepam, 242, 243
Dichotomous thinking, 165

Differentiation, 45–46
Disorientation, 26–27
Displacement, 41, 53, 54, 57, 152, 166–167
Dissociation, 168–169
Dissociative fugue, 16, 199, 205–206
Dissociative identity disorder, 195, 203
Distortion, 53, 152, 153, 166
Disulfiram, 260, 276
Dopamine, 70, 72, 73, 75, 76, 118
　antagonists, for treating Tourette's disorder, 259, 275–276
　receptor blockades, 253, 272, 274
Double-blind crossover studies, 253, 272
Down syndrome, 72
　dementia from, 113–114
Dreams, 43, 57
　and psychoanalysis, 165
　punishment, 54
Drug intoxication, 17
Durable power of attorney, 286, 291
Durham rule, 288, 292
Dyslexia, 80, 85
Dysthymic disorder, 10, 24, 72, 111, 176, 185–186, 191–192
Dystonia, 21, 62, 73
　neuroleptic-induced, 268, 281

E

Ebstein's anomaly, 277
Echolalia, 28
Echopraxia, 14, 28
Ego, 50, 51, 54
Egocentrism, 33, 48
Ego ideal, 50–51
Egomania, 16
Electroconvulsive therapy (ECT), 182, 189–191, 252, 271
Elimination half-life, of medication, 251, 254, 262, 270, 272, 277, 279
Encephalopathy
　chronic traumatic, 108, 123
　Wernicke's, 99, 117
Endorphins, 59, 70

Enuresis, 81, 87
　imipramine for treating, 266, 280
Epidural hematomas, 108, 122
Epilepsy, temporal lobe, 98, 116
Erikson, Erik, theories of, 34, 38, 41, 46–49, 52, 55
Erotomanic delusions, 131, 142
Exhibitionism, 219, 229
Exposure techniques, 160, 171, 173, 196, 204
Extinction, 154, 167, 168, 173

F

Factitious disorder, 100, 102, 110–111, 117, 119, 201–202, 217, 227–228
Failure to thrive, 36, 51
False negatives, 12, 26
Family intervention, 156, 169
Family therapy, 157, 158, 168, 170–171
Fetal alcohol syndrome, 81, 86
Fetishism, 219, 220, 229
　transvestic, 222
Flashbacks, from hallucinogen use, 239, 247
Flight of ideas, 16, 22, 26, 27
Flooding, 168
Fluoxetine, 258, 275, 279
Fluphenazine, 272, 275
Folie à deux, 28
Fragile X syndrome, 61, 72
Freud, Sigmund, 161, 163, 171
　and defense mechanisms, 52–53
　and dreams, 54, 57
　guidelines for psychotherapy, 159, 166, 172
　"Mourning and Melancholia" paper, 181, 189
　and primary processes, 37, 52, 165
　psychosexual development theories, 42, 44, 46, 47, 55–57
　structural theory of the mind, 41, 50–51, 55
　topographic model of the mind, 42, 54, 56–57

Index

Fromm-Reichmann, Frieda, theories of, 144–145
Frontal lobe tumors, 110
Frotteurism, 219, 220, 229
Fugue, 28
   dissociative, 16, 199, 205–206

G

GABA, 66, 76
   receptors for, 59, 70, 245, 265, 279
Gender dysphoria, 228
Gender identity, 40, 54, 218, 228
Gender identity disorder, 209, 222
Gender role, 40, 54
Generalized anxiety disorder (GAD), 115, 204, 206
Generativity vs. stagnation, 49
Genital stage, 55, 56
Gerstmann-Straussler syndrome, 115
Global Assessment of Functioning (GAF) scale, 191
Glucose, serum levels of, 17
Glutamate, 66
Goodpasture syndrome, 119
Grandiose delusion, 16
Grand mal seizures, 122
Group cohesion, 163

H

Habit reversal training, 159, 172
Half-life, of medication, 251, 254, 262, 270, 272, 277, 279
Hallucinations, 121
   from alcohol withdrawal, 243
   from anti-Parkinson's medication, 65, 75
   autoscopic, 137, 146
   from cocaine intoxication, 245
   in delusional disorder, 140
   explained, 7, 16, 17, 22, 143
   hypnagogic, 229
   with partial complex seizures, 95, 111, 113
   in schizophrenia, 139

Hallucinogens
   flashbacks from using, 239, 247
   LSD, 144
Haloperidol, 101, 118, 242, 272
   for treating Tourette's disorder, 259, 276
Haloperidol decanoate, 275
   and TD, 132, 142
Hippocampus, 66, 76
Histrionic personality disorder, 212, 224
HIV-associated dementia, 9, 23–24, 98, 116–117
Homosexuality, 222, 225
Humor, as defense mechanism, 157, 170
Huntington's disease, 69, 78, 96, 108, 113, 122, 191
   testing for, 8, 23
Hurler's syndrome, 72
Hyperprolactinemia, 118, 272
Hypersomnia, primary, 218, 219, 229
Hyperthyroidism, 106, 121
Hyperventilation, 97, 115
   paper-bag breathing technique for, 98, 116
Hypnagogic hallucinations, 229
Hypnosis, 149, 155, 163, 168–169
Hypoactive sexual disorder, 213, 224–225
Hypochondriasis, 110, 193, 196, 201, 204
Hypoglycemia, 17, 116
Hypothalamus, 66, 76
Hypothyroidism, 9, 23, 73, 116, 272–273, 278

I

Id, 50, 52
Idealization, 172
Ideas of reference, 1, 16, 22
Identification, 53, 152, 153, 166
Identity vs. role confusion, 48–49
Illusion, 2, 16, 17, 22
Imipramine, for treating enuresis, 266, 280

Impotence, 227
Imprinting, 44–45
Impulse control disorders, 207, 221
Incidence, disease, 26
Industry vs. inferiority, 45, 48
Infanticide, 143
Infantile neurosis, 44
Infantile sexuality, 57
Informed decisions, 285, 290
Inhalants, abuse of, 239, 246–247
Insanity defense, move to abolish, 292–293
Integrity vs. despair, 34, 48–49
Intellectualization, 23, 39, 53–54
Interpersonal psychotherapy, 159, 173
Interpersonal School of Thought, 181, 189
Interpretation, 155, 168
Intimacy vs. isolation, 49
Introjection, 53, 152, 166
Involuntary hospitalization, justification for, 284, 289
Irresistible impulse rule, 288, 292
Isolation, 23
Isolation of affect, 152, 159, 166, 172

J
Jung, Carl, concepts of, 34, 50, 151, 165

K
Kernberg, Otto, theories of, 161
Klein, Melanie, theories of, 46, 47, 55, 161
  Object Relation movement, 181, 189
Kleptomania, 221
Klüver-Bucy syndrome, 77
Kohlberg, Lawrence, concepts of, 46, 50
Kohut, Heinz, theories of, 32, 34, 35, 46–47, 49–51, 55, 151, 165, 179, 188
Koro, 136, 145
Korsakoff's syndrome, 74, 76, 103, 110, 116, 120
Kübler-Ross stages, 94, 112

L
Latency stage, 31, 45, 55
L-dopa, 60, 65, 70, 75
Legal insanity, 285, 290
Lesions
  of brain, 63, 67, 68, 74, 77
  of CNS, 113
Levodopa, 60, 65, 70, 75
Levothyroxine, 262, 278
Lithium, 145, 179, 188, 254, 272–273
  and birth defects, 261, 277
  half-life of, 262, 277
  for treating depression, 182, 190
  for treating mania, 177, 186, 267, 281
Long-term care, 25
Loose associations, 16, 27
Lycanthropy, 146
Lysergic acid diethylamide (LSD), 144

M
Magical thinking, 14, 28
Magnetic resonance imaging (MRI), 17, 23
Mahler, Margaret, theories of, 32, 45, 46
Major depression, 60, 61, 71, 73, 127, 139, 187
  and bereavement, 186
  and pancreatic cancer, 175, 185
Mal de ojo, 136, 145
Malingering, 111, 117, 119, 201, 228
Malpractice lawsuits, 283
  Four D's of, 289
  reasons for, 286, 291
Mamillary bodies, 66, 76
Mania, 16
Marijuana, 238, 246
  use during pregnancy, 86
MDMA, 239, 247
Melatonin, 71
Mens rea elements, 288, 292
Mental retardation (MR), 19, 90
  and ADHD, 79, 85
  inherited, 72
  moderate, 4, 18

Mental status examinations, 3, 18, 26
Meperidine, intoxication from, 232, 242
Minnesota Multiphasic Personality Inventory (MMPI), 6, 191
MMPI, 20–21
M'Naghten rule, 292–293
Model Penal Code, 293
Monoamine oxidase inhibitors (MAOIs), 61, 72–73, 190, 192, 206, 269, 273
  interaction with sympathomimetic agents, 265, 279–280
Multi-infarct dementia, 5, 19, 96, 110, 114, 191
Multiple sclerosis (MS), 113, 194, 202
Multiple transference, 164
Munchausen syndrome, 88, 119
Mutism
  in catatonic schizophrenia, 140
  selective, 83, 88–89
Myoglobin, urine levels of, 17

N
Naloxone, 232, 242
Narcissistic personality disorder, 171, 217, 227
Narcolepsy, 70, 218, 219, 228–229
  medication for, 260, 277
  and REM sleep, 208, 222, 229, 280
Necrophilia, 229
Neologisms, 16
Nervios, 136, 145
Neuroleptic malignant syndrome (NMS), 17, 125, 138, 266, 273, 280
Neuroleptics
  and akathisia, 249, 269
  and dystonia, 168, 281
  potency-level differences of, 272, 279
Neuropeptides, 66, 76
Neurotransmitters, 66, 76
Neutrality, as Freudian concept, 172
Nicotine dependence, treatment for, 236, 246
Night terrors, 64, 75

Nihilism, 28
Nocturnal myoclonus, 111–112
Nocturnal penile tumescence (NPT), 216, 226–227
Non-benzodiazepine antianxiolytics, 200, 206
Non-REM (NREM) sleep, 64, 75
Norepinephrine, 66, 72, 73, 75, 76, 271
Normal-pressure hydrocephalus (NPH), 99, 117

O
Object constancy, 45, 46, 51–52
Object permanence, 37, 51
Object relation theory, 161
Obsessions, 28, 202
Obsessive-compulsive disorder (OCD), 173, 194, 195, 199, 202, 205, 206, 270
Obsessive-compulsive personality disorder, 3, 18, 75, 171, 212, 224
Occipital lobe tumors, 105, 121
Oedipal stage, 42, 55
Olanzapine, 131, 142, 270, 273, 279
Operant conditioning, 168
Opiate
  intoxication, 232, 241–242
  use during pregnancy, 86
  withdrawal, 231, 235, 242, 244
Oppositional defiant disorder (ODD), 80, 85–86, 90
Oral contraceptives, and depression, 180, 188
Oral stage, 44, 55, 56
Orientation, 3, 18
Outpatient commitment, 25

P
Pain disorder, 102, 118–119
Pancreatic carcinoma, 103, 120
Panic attacks, 17, 193, 201
Panic disorder, 115, 193, 201, 206
  cognitive treatment of, 158, 171
Paranoia, 4, 18–19

Paranoid personality disorder, 214, 225–226
Paraphilias, 229
Parapraxes, 57
Parkinson's disease, 93, 111, 142, 281–282
  and clozapine, 261, 277
  ECT for treating, 189, 271
Pathological gambling, 207, 221
Perception, 28
Performance anxiety, 204, 277
Periodic limb movement disorder, 218, 228
Perphenazine, 126, 138
Perseveration, 13, 16, 26, 27
Personality disorders, 202, 209, 222–223
  lifetime prevalence of, 213, 225
  therapy for, 148, 162–163, 171
Personalization, 165
Phallic stage, 55, 56
Phencyclidine (PCP), 144, 233, 235, 236, 242, 244–245
  symptoms of intoxication, 144, 233, 235, 242, 244–245
  treatment of intoxication, 236, 245
Phenobarbital, 278
Phenothiazines, 273–274
Pheochromocytoma, 107, 122
Phobias
  specific, 196, 198, 203–205
  treatment for, 168, 196, 197, 204, 206
Phototherapy, 263, 278
Piaget, Jean, theories of, 32, 42, 46, 47, 50–51, 55
Piblokto, 146
Pick's disease, 91, 109, 116
Piloerection, 241
Pituitary gland tumors, 105, 121
Placebos, 102, 119, 253, 272
Polydipsia, psychogenic, 135, 145
Polypharmacy, 104, 120
Polysomnography, 227, 229

Poor metabolizers, 263, 278
Positive transference, 151, 166
Positron emission tomography (PET), 183, 191
Postcardiotomy delirium, 104, 121
Postpartum blues, 175, 176, 185
Postpartum depression, 178, 187
Postpartum psychosis, 133, 143–144
Poststroke depression, 178, 186–187
Posttraumatic stress disorder (PTSD), 143, 199, 205
  medication for, 264, 278–279
Potentiation, defined, 240, 248
Practicing, 46
Prader-Willi syndrome, 61, 71–72
Preconscious, 57
Prednisone, 187, 274
Pregnancy
  drug and alcohol use during, 81, 86–87
  and medication side effects, 257, 261, 275, 277
  and restless legs syndrome, 208, 222
Premature ejaculation, 156, 169
Premenstrual dysphoric disorder (PMDD), 104, 120, 209, 223
Premenstrual syndrome (PMS), 104, 120
Prevalence, 12, 25–26
Priapism, and trazodone, 251, 269, 271
Primary gain, 41, 55, 100, 117
Primary prevention, 11, 25
Primary processes, 37, 43, 52, 57
Principle of beneficence, 286, 291
Privileged communication, 285, 290
Projection, 17, 22, 53, 152, 153, 166, 172
Projective identification, 152, 153, 166
Prolactin, 101, 103, 107, 118, 120, 122
Propranolol, 210, 223, 277
Psychic determinism, 55
Psychoanalysis, 157, 158, 171
  classical, 165
Psychological tests, 6, 20

Psychotherapy
  brief individual, 157, 158, 170
  client-centered, 150, 164
  supportive, 150, 164
Purging, 92, 110, 216, 227
Pyromania, 80, 86, 221

R
Rabbit syndrome, 268, 282
Raphe nuclei, 63, 74
Rapid eye movement (REM) sleep, 60, 61, 70, 71, 73, 75, 89, 191
  and narcolepsy, 208, 222, 276
  and NPT, 226
  suppression by antidepressants, 265, 280
Rapprochement, 32, 46
Rating scales, 20
Rationalization, 23, 54
Reaction formation, 22, 38, 53, 152, 166, 172
Reactive attachment disorder, 82, 88
Reframing, 168
Reinforcement, 154, 167
Relative risk, 26
Relaxation techniques, 165
Repression, 54, 152, 166
Resistance, 149, 163
Restless legs syndrome, 208, 222
Rett's disorder, 2, 17, 72, 115
Rogers, Carl, 164
Rubella, 65, 76

S
Sangue dormido, 145
Scatologia, 219, 229
Schizoaffective disorder, 19, 129, 130, 140–142
Schizoid personality disorder, 222
Schizophrenia, 5, 19, 21, 26, 27, 70, 134, 144, 169, 222, 226
  disorganized, 128, 139, 140
  inheritance of, 126, 139

Schizophrenia (*Cont.*):
  medication for, 141, 142
  and polydipsia, 135, 145
  suicide risk of, 132, 143
Schizophreniform disorder, 127, 139, 143
Schizotypal personality disorder, 208, 221–222
School phobia, 89
SCIDR, 20
SCL-90-R, 20
Seasonal affective disorder, 183, 184, 192
Seasonal circadian rhythm, 60, 71
Seasonal depression, phototherapy for, 263, 278
Secondary gain, 55, 100, 117
Secondary prevention, 12, 25
Secondary revision, 54, 57
Seizures
  absence, 111
  during clozapine treatment, 263, 278
  grand mal, 122
  nonepileptic, 9, 24
  partial complex, 64, 74, 93, 95, 111, 113
  tonic-clonic, 120
Selective abstraction, 165
Selective mutism, 83, 88–89
Self-Psychology, 46–47, 49–50, 165
Sensate focus exercises, 156, 169
Sensitivity, 26
Separation-individuation theory, 32, 45–46
Serotonin, 65, 72, 73, 76, 190, 273
  and aggression, 64, 75
Serotonin syndrome, 255, 273
Sexual identity, 40, 54
Shared belief system, 163–164
Sleep apnea, 94, 111
Sleep deprivation, 179, 187
Sleep terror disorder, 89

Sleepwalking disorder, 207, 221
Social phobia, 11, 25, 197, 198, 204, 206
  contrasted with avoidant personality disorder, 226
Somatization, 152, 166
Somatization disorder, 117–119, 199, 202, 205
Spitz, Renée, studies of, 36, 51
Splitting, 147, 161
Squeeze technique, 169
SSRI discontinuation syndrome, 264, 279
SSRIs, 190, 200, 206, 269–271, 273, 276
Start-and-stop technique, 169
Steroids
  adrenocortical, 256, 274
  anabolic, abuse of, 232, 241
Stevens-Johnson syndrome, 273
Stranger anxiety, 36–37, 51
Structural theory, 57
Stuttering, 84, 89–90
Subarachnoid hemorrhage, 122–123
Subdural hematomas, 92, 110, 122
Sublimation, 38, 53, 152, 166, 171–172
Substance abuse, defined, 240, 247–248
Substance-induced mood disorder, 95, 112–113, 178, 187
Substance P, 66
Suggestibility, 155, 168–169
Suicide, 5, 20, 143
  and malpractice claims, 291
  in mood disorders, 179, 187
Sullivan, Harry Stack, theories of, 37, 52, 144, 173
  Interpersonal School of Thought, 181, 189
Superego, 35, 50–51
Supportive psychotherapy, 150, 164
Suppression, 166, 170

SVIB, 20
Symbiosis, 45
Sympathomimetic agents, interaction with MAOIs, 265, 279–280
Synesthesia, 17, 21–22
Syphilis, tertiary, 107, 122

T

Tangentiality, 26, 27
Tarasoff-I decision, 286, 290–291
Tarasoff-II decision, 287, 291
Tardive dyskinesia (TD), 125, 138–139, 142, 273, 274, 282, 290
Temperament, 34, 45, 49
Temporal lobe epilepsy (TLE), 98, 116
Temporal lobe tumors, 106, 121
Tertiary prevention, 25
Thematic apperception test (TAT), 6, 21
Theory of the mind, 228
"The Principles of Medical Ethics with Annotations Especially Applicable to Psychiatry," 292
Thiamine deficiency, 63, 74, 76, 116, 117, 243
Thioridazine, 279
Thought broadcasting, 28
Thought insertion, 27
Tics, 81, 87
Time-out, 167
Token economy, 157, 170
Tolerance, defined, 240, 248
Topographic model, 42, 54, 56–57
Tourette's syndrome, 81, 87
  medication for, 259, 275–276
Trail-making test, 21
Trance states, 22
Transference, 147, 161–162
  exploitation by psychiatrists, 292
  multiple, 164
  positive, 151, 166
Transference neurosis, 148, 162

Transitional objects, 33, 47
Transvestic fetishism, 215, 222, 226
Trazodone, and priapism, 251, 269, 271
Tricyclic antidepressants (TCAs), 190, 200, 206, 251, 269–271, 273
  anticholinergic side effects from, 258, 275
  cardiac effects from, 267, 281
  overdose of, 257, 274
Trust vs. mistrust, 48
Twins, studies on, 175, 185
Tyramine, 72

U

Uncomplicated bereavement, 176, 186
Unconscious, 57
Universalization, 149, 163
Unwanted treatment, 284, 290

V

Vaginismus, 215, 226
Validation, 163
Validity, of studies, 26
Valproate, side effects of, 257, 275
VDRL, 107, 122
Vineland Adaptive Behavior Scales, 21

Violence
  from Amok, 145
  signs of impending, 19
  and Tarasoff-II decision, 291
Vitamin B_{12} deficiency, 109
VMA, urine, 107, 122

W

Waxy flexibility, 21
Wernicke-Korsakoff syndrome, 116
Wernicke's encephalopathy, 99, 117
Weschler Adult Intelligence Scale (WAIS), 191
Weschler Intelligence Scale for Children (WISC), 21
Williams' syndrome, 72
Wilson's disease, 97, 114–115
Windigo, 145
Winnicott, D.W., concepts of, 33, 47–48
Wisconsin card sorting test, 20
Wish fulfillment, 55
Withdrawal, defined, 240, 248
Withdrawal dyskinesia, 138
Word salad, 26

Z

Zoophilia, 229